GREAT MEN with sick brains

& other essays

Bengt Ljunggren, MD, PhD

Published by
American Association of
Neurological Surgeons
Park Ridge, Illinois

Library of Congress Catalog Number: 89-81019
ISBN: 0-9624246-0-9

This publication is published under the auspices of the Publications Committee of the American Association of Neurological Surgeons (AANS). However, this should not be construed as indicating endorsement or approval of the views presented, by the AANS, or by its committees, commissions, affiliates, or staff.

Robert H. Wilkins, MD, Chairman
AANS Publications Committee

Gabrielle J. Loring, Publications Production Manager

AANS1M1189

Contents

Preface

William Macewen (1848-1924), Victor Horsley (1857-1916), and Francesco Durante (1845-1934) are well-recognized pioneers of brain surgery. There were, however, other less recognized workers in this new specialty.

While it is commonly believed that surgery of the nervous system was perfected and introduced as a specialty in the first decade of this century by the American Harvey Cushing (1869-1939), it should be noted that there were many pioneers in central Europe and in the Nordic countries. Wilhelm Wagner (1848-1900) from Königshütte in Upper Silesia was the inventor of the osteoplastic flap so necessary for exploration of the brain. Vilhelm Magnus (1871-1929) from Oslo worked in parallel with and quite independently from the great American neurosurgeons; his operative results in no way fell short of Cushing's. Magnus' impressions of American neurosurgery in the year 1928 are included in this book.

This book is aimed at neuroscientists with an interest in the lives and accomplishments of some pioneers in neurology and surgical neurology as well as the lives and accomplishments (good or bad) of some of their more renowned patients. I also have taken the liberty to include a more unusual case of a foreign body introduced into the brain with a survey of the literature on this matter (see Chapter 9).

Permission to reproduce excerpts from previously published articles was kindly granted by the publishers of *Surgical Neurology* (Chapters 1, 6, 8, 9), *British Journal of Neurosurgery* (Chapter 2), *Journal of Neurosurgery* (Chapter 5), and *Neurosurgery* (Chapter 7). I had great help during many years from innumerable persons all over the world. There are some who I would specifically like to mention: my German colleague Michael Buchfelder (Chapter 1), my colleagues Harald Fodstad and Kristian Kristiansen from Norway, Ib Sögaard from Denmark and Tapio Törmä from Finland (Chapter 2), my Swedish colleagues Bo Norrving and Ido Leden (Chapter 4), Ms. Anne Waugh and Ms. Birgitta Ermståhl, who offered excellent secretarial work, and last but not least, my brother Magnus Ljunggren (all chapters and especially Chapters 3 and 4).

Chapter 1

The Pioneers Who Laid the Cornerstones for Routine Opening of the Cranial Vault

Many surgical approaches have been proposed to facilitate exposure of lesions in the skull base region with a minimum of brain retraction. The approach to the circle of Willis and its environs with the microsurgical techniques now routinely used is pterional. This implies that a small skull flap is raised with pterion—the craniometric point located underneath the temporalis muscle and formed by the junction of the frontal, parietal, and temporal bones with the great sphenoid wing—in the center at the base of the flap. Additional drilling down the sphenoid ridge allows a low basal exposure along the skull base.

Equipped with the microsurgical instruments of today, the pterional approach to skull base lesions is an easy and most natural procedure for the experienced neurosurgeon. Yet, there is a fascinating historical background that forms the basis for opening of the cranial vault. Also, there are some distinguished pioneers who each have made a major contribution in the development of the access to intracranial lesions.

Wilhelm Wagner (1848-1900)

Virtually unknown to modern neurosurgeons, Wilhelm Wagner (1848-1900) was an industrious, versatile, and courageous surgeon with brilliant surgical talent. He not only devoted his skill to cranial surgery but also took a keen interest in spinal injuries. A respected internist, Wagner gained an international reputation as an eminent botanist.

Following studies on human cadavers 100 years ago, this German pioneer developed the technique of raising a bone flap from the cranial vault that is kept attached to the covering soft tissue during intracranial surgery. This ingenious innovation, the osteoplastic flap, was a significant contribution to neurological surgery. A century later, modified techniques of Wagner's original approach are still discussed in leading journals of the neurosciences.

Early Career

Wilhelm Wagner, the son of a pastor, was born on January 14, 1848, in the small village of Wohnbach in Hesse, Germany. At the age of 16, he began his medical studies at the University of Giessen, which he then continued in Marburg. He attended lectures by the clinical teachers Heusinger, Rose, Dohrn, and Benecke. He received his Doctor of Medicine in 1869 after having written a doctoral thesis, "Ueber die Percussion des Magens nach Auftreibung mit Kohlensäure. Ein Beitrag zur Anatomie und physikalischen Diagnostik."

He then worked as a doctor at a spa in Bad Nauheim but was soon, like his compatriot and colleague Ernst von Bergmann, ordered to participate as a physician in the Franco-Prussian War in 1870. During war service Wagner was detached to work in the reserve infirmary in nearby Friedberg. With self-sacrificing ardor, he devoted all his time to treating injured soldiers from both sides.

After the war, he stayed in Friedberg, not far from his parental home. Here he married Marie Herzberger, who by sympathizing with his ambitions supported him in all his ventures and created a secure background against which his work could proceed and develop. Their marriage was harmonious and was to last for 27 years.

Within a short time Wagner became well-known in Friedberg as a skillful and capable young doctor; soon his good reputation spread all over Hesse. He did not receive training in operations from any master of surgery. Yet, as a self-trainee, he soon learned how to perform operations with an increasing degree of difficulty. He also found time to follow the literature in medicine. Besides a busy practice, he continuously presented interesting reports, articles, and reviews related to all branches of the art of healing. For this industrious worker with a sharp intellect and an insatiable thirst for more knowledge, peaceful Friedberg soon became too limited.

When in 1877 Wagner learned of a vacant position in a hospital in Königshütte, a small town in a mining district in Upper Silesia, he applied for the vacancy, was accepted, and moved. In Königshütte, which in 1880 had a population of 27,631 inhabitants, Wagner came to stay for the rest of his life. While Ernst von Bergmann in 1882 was appointed professor of surgery in Berlin and became one of the great surgeons of Europe, highly regarded by such famous contemporaries as Volkmann and Theodor Billroth, Wagner refrained from an academic career. Instead, he devoted his lifework to helping the people in this mining region who were stricken with illness or accidents. It was here, in this muddy and grey corner of the world, that he came to accomplish so much.

Master Surgeon in Königshütte

In Königshütte Wagner developed into a master surgeon with a particular interest focused on treatment of cranial and spinal injuries. Despite a heavy daily clinical practice, he incessantly studied and followed new books and journals not only in the field of surgery but also in general medicine and other related branches. Wagner was beloved by his patients, for he radiated goodness and security; he became renowned in the whole of Silesia not only for his supreme surgical skill but also for his great knowledge and good results in the treatment of nonsurgical diseases.

He soon started to write his own publications. Wilhelm Wagner published important contributions on a variety of problems primarily of surgical interest but also some related to general medicine. His work on the treatment of empyema was translated into English and appeared in the *Medical and Surgical Reporter* in 1881. His publications on the management of complicated skull fractures and clinical diagnosis and operative management of epidural hematomas are still masterpieces.

Injuries of the Spine and Spinal Cord

Besides his interest in surgery of intracranial lesions, Wilhelm Wagner also showed an interest in problems related to orthopedics and affections of the spine. He described the practical value of Sayre's plaster corset for the correction of kyphosis and scoliosis and for the treatment of spinal fractures. These interests developed from the beginning of his work in Königshütte in 1877.

In 1884 at the 13th Congress of the German Society of Surgery in Berlin, Wagner presented a paper on cervical spine luxation fractures that included a case of odontoid peg fracture and another of a compression fracture resulting in a Brown-Séquard syndrome. He proceeded on this subject and the following year published his experiences of luxation fractures in the cervical spine. *Die Verletzungen der Wirbelsäule und des Rückenmarks* (*The Injuries of the Spine and the Spinal Cord*) was to become his most remarkable volume, written in close collaboration with his former pupil, Paul Stolper, who later worked in Breslau (Wroclaw) as a general surgeon. In their voluminous book consisting of 564 pages and many illustrations, the authors cover the whole subject of anatomy and physiology of the spine and spinal cord and discuss the pathology and symptomatology of spine and spinal cord injuries. However, the most original part consists of a compilation of their own experience by presenting numerous illustrative cases that are described in detail.

They state their principal and basic intention: "The personal experiences of injuries of the vertebral column that are documented in this publication are based on the material obtained over a period of about 20 years from the Miners' Guild Infirmary in Königshütte, and on that of my [Wagner's] practice as a consultant and court expert. There are more than 500 relevant observations. The most instructive part of these cases, however, are those treated exclusively in the hospital during the last 15 years. All those who died there underwent autopsy. There are clinical records available in the vast majority of these cases and hence the main data as compiled in our table are instructive enough to justify their presentation, particularly since up to now no author, except for Theodor Kocher, has reported more extensively on any personal material. We have not presented the observations from our consultant practice here, since the cases dealt with in such a practice have already undergone some selection. Admittedly there are, among these, rarer and frequently interesting observations, but we were primarily interested in the prognosis as estimated from average data. The clinical data obtained from the catchment area of a Miners' Guild Infirmary in Upper Silesia allows one to draw particularly reliable conclusions since all healed patients with some reduction of the capability to earn their livelihood present themselves again at their original sanatorium for check-ups or for collecting their disability benefits."

The therapeutic approach of the authors to spine and spinal cord injuries was predominantly conservative. Luxation fractures, however, required correction. The avoidance of precisely described secondary complications was held to be the major goal. The authors held a reserved view regarding operative intervention. A few sentences deal with the prospective value that x-ray investigation might eventually attain in these kind of injuries, a farsighted view at the time. That Wagner's knowledge of spinal injuries was highly regarded is demonstrated by the fact that professor von Bergmann in Berlin, to support his own view, consulted Wagner as a court expert in a case of spinal injury.

Wilhelm Wagner at the Top

Wagner's ceaseless work both as a practicing surgeon and as a busy writer led to his attaining a wide reputation all over his home country. He was able to transform his rather small institution into an exemplary hospital for diseases and accidental injuries. He also had to overcome a lot of nonmedical problems. When he had started his work in Königshütte in 1877, he was the only doctor in the hospital and was offered a permanent assistant only in 1882. He had to solve the logistical problems of heating and accommodation; apart from the acute treatment of injuries, some rehabilitation also was made possible within this institution.

Wagner became protocolist and later chairman of the local Medical Association of the Industrial District of Upper Silesia and joined the Medical Association of Silesia. His efforts to improve the economic situation of the medical profession stemmed from these activities and fall among his major merits. In the German Society of Surgery, the doctor from the small town in Upper Silesia was a member for many years and occupied a prominent seat.

Apart from his vast professional engagements, he was also a well-known botanist who corresponded with many centers in all parts of the world. Wagner's herbarium was as perfect and complete as its master.

Wagner also engaged in local politics, founded a recreation center in Bad Gonczalkowitz for the miners and foundry workers, and a sanatorium for victims of pulmonary diseases in Loslau. He was among those who instituted a local modern secondary school for girls in Königshütte, where he served as a trustee for many years. He was honored on many occasions. His love for mountains and nature led to his being appointed an honorary member of the Carpathian Society. Later a peak in the Tatra Mountains was named after him—the Wagnerspitze. First given the title "Geheimer Sanitätsrat," he was later declared professor in 1894.

Professor Wagner suffered more or less chronically from an infection that he had acquired during surgery many years before. He sometimes had to leave to take a cure in Tarasp, Bormio, or Badgastein. In 1897, he had to operate on his own wife with a most disastrous result: his beloved life-companion died. One might compare this tragedy with the staggering blow that fell on Harvey Cushing 30 years later when he lost General Leonard Wood in an unexpected hemorrhage following surgery for a recurrent meningioma (see Chapter 5).

Following this tragedy Professor Wagner increasingly became introverted and taciturn until his death of a stroke on August 6, 1900.

In 1908 the local authorities erected a monument consisting of a metal plaque bearing Wagner's portrait and the inscription "Aliis inserviendo consumor" (Fig 1) in a central place. A square in the main street and a street adjoining the hospital area were named after him. In 1921, when Königshütte following the negotiations of Versailles came under Polish government (at first renamed to Królewska Huta, and as from 1934 to Chozzóh or Chorzów), the stone monument was moved to the hospital area and the plaque of Wagner was replaced by a plaque bearing the portrait of the Polish doctor Andrzej Mielecki. There the monument still stands with the plaque

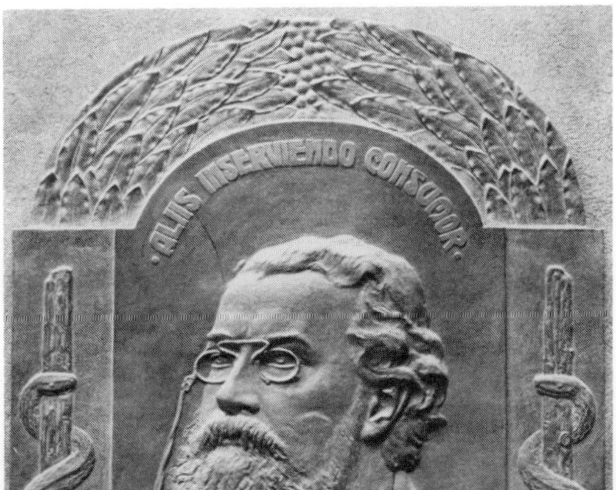

Figure 1: *Wagner's memorial in Königshütte (later Królewska Huta, now Chorzów, Poland) in Upper Silesia, which consisted of a metal plate carrying his portrait and the inscription "Aliis inserviendo consumor" (I am consumed by devotion to others).*

of Mielecki, who back in the early 1920s had fought hard for a boundary line that incorporated Königshütte with Poland and not with Germany.

In summary, due to the frequent political changes in this region, Wagner became a forgotten pioneer and his most important contributions to neurosurgery appear not to have been recognized by the modern neurosurgical community.

Wagner's Pioneering Osteoplastic Craniotomy

The major achievement for which Wilhelm Wagner should be remembered by posterity is his careful study of human cadavers that led to his descriptive paper on intraoperative raising of a cranial vault bone flap in 1889. Wagner's flap is kept attached to the temporal muscle and aponeurosis and may subsequently be repositioned following intracranial surgery. In his important article, Wagner suggested that his procedure—the method of osteoplastic craniotomy—should be of value not only for removing hematomas "arising from the dura" but also for extirpation of intracranial tumors and brain abscesses and to allow cortical resection for epilepsy.

It should be remembered that Julius Wolff, following experimental work on rabbits in 1863, had shown that osteoplastic techniques were possible. Wagner knew Wolff personally and was aware of the latter's pioneering experimental studies. He also mentioned this in a later study from 1891 in which he described the successful temporary elevation of large flaps in two children with chronic sequelae of brain injury and epileptic seizures. In this paper, Wagner states that he had discussed the question of priority with his friend Julius Wolff in "a most friendly manner." Wolff had performed his experimental animal studies but had not pursued the matter further. It was Wagner who, following studies for several years on human cadavers, had the imagination, surgical skill, and courage to transfer the method to living humans.

Wagner's First Report

In his first report, Wagner made it clear that in his opinion "the removal of healthy osseous cranial vault is a mutilating operation because the brain is deprived of its natural protection and, although firm scar tissue may develop and offer some protection, many such patients are forced to have their bony defect covered by an artificial protective shield." He continued his opinion:

> "I have for some time been trying to find a method through studies on cadavers by which one could resect a part of the cranial vault of the required size so that it can be completely removed from its place, but remains connected to the soft tissue, so that it can be reimplanted after the operative procedure without nutritional disturbances and so that healing is secured.
>
> "After various attempts, I came to employ the following method: After an incision in the shape of the Greek omega, the soft tissue of the respective cranial region is incised down to the periosteum. As soon as the flap has retracted, it is compressed against the cranial vault and a periosteal incision is made along its

margin which thus runs 1/2 to 1 cm within and parallel to the first incision. Then, the whole thickness of the bone is chiseled along the curve of this inner omega-shaped incision while in the limbs only one groove is chiseled, which increases in size from inside to outside. In the limbs two small chisels are inserted and, without traumatising the overlying soft-tissue flap, the bony connection is chiseled through subcutaneously.

"Subsequently, it is quite easy to elevate the piece of bone which is outlined from the curve of the omega and to flap it back together with the (attached) soft tissues parallel to the limbs of the omega. Between these limbs, the bone flap together with all the soft tissues attached to it remains connected to the remaining cover of the cranium by a pedicle of at least 3 cm width.

"The flapped-back piece is then simply reinserted into its former place. The soft tissue flap, which due to the difference in the soft tissue and bone incisions overlaps the latter for about 1 cm, is carefully sutured again, as are the limbs of the omega after drainage of the angles. The piece of bone always fits very well into the gap especially if the small edges of the inner table, which remain in the bone gap, are preserved in order to prevent the resected part from sinking inwards. After I had sufficiently convinced myself of the easy feasibility of the operation through experiments on cadavers, I recently had the opportunity to perform this on a living individual."

Subsequently Wagner presented an elegant description of a 27-year-old man who had sustained a severe head injury resulting in fractures of the base of the skull associated with symptoms of an expanding intracranial mass lesion. Certainly he was aware of the results of the meticulous experiments carried out by von Bergmann in Berlin on the cardiovascular and respiratory effect of increased intracranial pressure (ICP). He observed the phenomenon (now often referred to as the Cushing reflex, although von Bergmann had described it long before Cushing), i.e. increasing systolic and pulse pressure as well as bradycardia, the dreaded signs of rapidly increasing ICP frequently leading to cerebral herniations and midbrain and medullary compression.

He consequently decided to evacuate the epidural hematoma he suspected that the patient harbored. Surgery was undertaken on the second day following the cranial trauma. Prior to surgery the patient was in a poor condition. Following elevation of a temporal bone flap, Wagner had no difficulties in evacuating a large epidural hematoma. After surgery it was obvious that the ICP normalized. The patient, however, deteriorated and died 24 hours after surgery. At autopsy Wagner found no signs of disturbed nutrition in the omega-shaped flap in the temporal region that he had raised to allow evacuation of the hematoma, of which nothing remained. He concluded that his osteoplastic method was an easy procedure that resulted in a good exposure of tears in the middle meningeal artery branches in the middle cranial fossa.

Successful Evacuation of Epidural Hematoma via the Osteoplastic Flap

It was not until 1895 that Wagner was able to publish two further cases of successful evacuation of epidural hematomas through his osteoplastic flap. Wagner's original report

"Two cases of hematoma of the dura mater cured by temporary resection of the cranial vault" stated: "Although, since my first publication on the temporary resection of the cranial vault, this operation has now come to be so frequently carried out that it has more or less replaced the actual trepanation (if by this one understands the permanent resection of a piece of the osseous cranial vault) it seems that to date it has hardly been used for the evacuation of hematomas of the dura mater. I have at least been able to localize only one such case, that of Dr. Stenzel, who had a case with a successful outcome. Temporary resection of the cranial vault offers infinite advantages in comparison to craniectomy. In particular, one may further enlarge the opening as was done in my cases. One is much more certain of finding and occluding the source of the bleeding via this procedure. The ligation or suturing of tears in the middle meningeal artery is in any case particularly easy when such a lot of space is available. The same would have applied to the transverse sinus, which was successfully repaired in my second case. A further appreciable advantage is that when the source of bleeding is not immediately found, one is able to tamponade and to remove the tampon after several days and examine the interior of the cranial cavity again in order to see whether the hemorrhage has definitely stopped or if rebleeding has occurred, etc.

"In our case, after six days two minor branches of the meningeal artery still had to be ligated. I think that such small vessel injury in addition to the rupture of a larger one, may not only result from the force of the impact itself but may also result from the detachment of the dura from the cranial vault by a rapidly expanding extravasate.

"In his case, Stenzel also had to reraise the skin and bone flap since he could not find the source of bleeding and he had to insert a tampon. Such reraising of the flap is not harmful and may possibly even be recommended."

Wagner preferred to work with hammer and chisels and did not favor the use of rotating saws used by other surgeons of that time. Like Wagner, von Bergmann was particularly interested in surgery of the head and objected strongly to the use of chisel and hammer to open the skull, a technique with which Wagner obviously was very familiar and which in his hand had no adverse effects. In his 1880 book, von Bergmann already rejected Wagner's technique and fashioned his flaps by using drills and saws; the flexible Gigli's saw was not yet known by him. The adverse effects from hammer blows, Verhämmerung, experienced by many surgeons of the time were obviously due to a too traumatic technique. Wagner repeatedly stated that he never encountered such adverse effects from hammering, although he had "carefully looked out for them."

French Admiration of Wagner's Pioneering Work

In 1891, Professor Jean Toison ("professeur à la Faculté libre de Lille" in France) described his use of a chain saw to divide the skull bone between burr holes from within outward to facilitate raising of osteoplastic flaps. He offered a high estimation of Wagner's pioneering operation on October 1, 1889, and even included him in the title of his study. Toison's saw could replace hammer and chisels but was fairly clumsy; therefore, it was not used much.

Leonardo Gigli and His Cranial Saw

In 1894, Leonardo Gigli from Florence had described his simple yet ingenious instrument for sawing up bone; the tool has come to bear his name—the Gigli saw. Originally Gigli invented it in order to facilitate symphysiotomy in obstetrical surgery. He finished his original report emphasizing that one dozen saws could be obtained from the Hermann Härtel Company in Breslau at the price of three German marks and an additional 40 pfennigs for stamp expenses to any foreign country. In a later report (1897), Gigli recommended his saw for all kinds of bone resection "with the exception of course of skull bone" ("abgesehen natürlich denjenigen an der Hirnschale").

It was Professor Alfred Karol Obalinski (Fig 2), at the Jagiellonian University of Cracow in Galicia (geographically not far away from Königshütte in Upper Silesia), the haven of Polish culture at the time although under the government of Vienna, who described the use of the Gigli saw for cranial trepanations in 1897.

Obalinski had intended to present his innovation at the International Congress of Medicine in Moscow in August 1897 but—probably for political reasons—he had been prevented from traveling to Russia and instead published this major contribution in the *Centralblatt für Chirurgie* later the same year. In Moscow, instead, Monsieur Le Docteur E. Doyen demonstrated his procedure to perform craniectomy for professors Kocher (Berne), Czerny (Heidelberg), Simpson (Edinburgh), von Bergmann (Berlin), Sklifassowski (St. Petersburg), and some more distinguished surgeons (Fig 3).

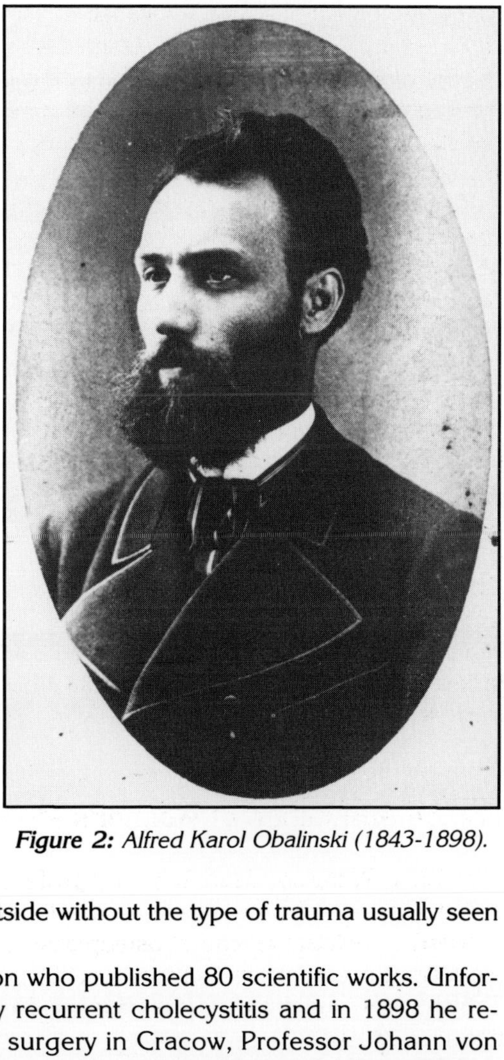

Figure 2: *Alfred Karol Obalinski (1843-1898).*

In his paper, Obalinski stated that it had struck him that the flexible Gigli saw should be ideal to introduce between burr holes using a slightly bended cannula as an inserter. He emphasized that the use of the Gigli saw permits the most cautious sawing up of the skull bone from the inside to the outside without the type of trauma usually seen from the use of hammer and chisel.

Professor Obalinski was an eminent surgeon who published 80 scientific works. Unfortunately, he was plagued for several years by recurrent cholecystitis and in 1898 he requested the help of the former professor of surgery in Cracow, Professor Johann von Mikulicz-Radecki in Breslau. The latter came to rescue his old friend and compatriot in surgery but the subsequent operation ended in a terrible disaster, that is, Professor Obalinski died due to surgical failure at the age of 55.

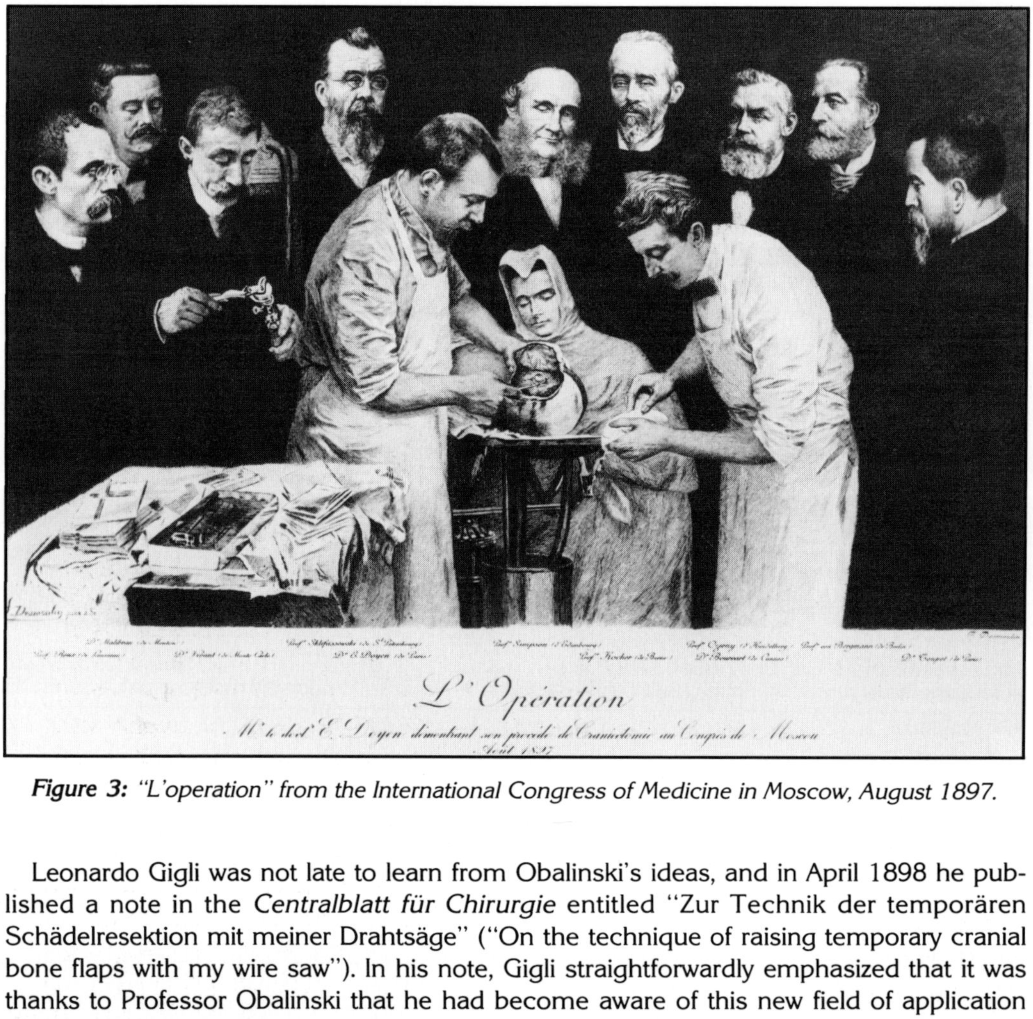

Figure 3: *"L'operation" from the International Congress of Medicine in Moscow, August 1897.*

Leonardo Gigli was not late to learn from Obalinski's ideas, and in April 1898 he published a note in the *Centralblatt für Chirurgie* entitled "Zur Technik der temporären Schädelresektion mit meiner Drahtsäge" ("On the technique of raising temporary cranial bone flaps with my wire saw"). In his note, Gigli straightforwardly emphasized that it was thanks to Professor Obalinski that he had become aware of this new field of application for his wire saw. He also described a probe or inserter for his saw between burr holes: "Die grösste Schwierigkeit der Technik der Kraniektomi mit meiner Säge besteht darin, letztere unter den Knochen des Schädels durchzuführen, und zwar ohne Ausübung von Druck und ohne Verletzung der Hirnhäute. Ich habe zu dem Zweck eine Art rinnenförmiger Sonde ausführen lassen. . . ." (The major difficulty in performing a craniectomy with my saw is associated with the introduction of it under the skull bone without exertion of pressure on the underlying cerebral membranes. For this purpose I have designed a special curved probe. . . .)

Wagner's Description of His Osteoplastic Procedure in 1895

Gigli's technical innovation—to become applied to cranial surgery thanks to his Polish colleague Obalinski—was probably not known to Wagner when in 1895 he described the technical problems associated with the procedure of performing an osteoplastic craniotomy:

"As to the performance of the temporary resection of the cranial vault, during recent years I have always had to utilize the chisel as in both of these cases. The craniotomy saw described by Salzer is, as designed by Thürriegel, too fragile to be used for proper work, as are the simple rotating saws. Even less adequate is the saw mentioned by Arendt which protects the dura from being torn off and which requires much more force than an ordinary rotating saw. I saw recently at Mikulicz's a saw constructed by Härtel in Breslau, in which the weak spiral which transmits the power to the actual rotating saw is replaced by a bar broken three times. Mikulicz is very satisfied with it. Sonnenburg also highly praises the saw which he himself described. Unfortunately, I have not yet seen it. Since I am using stronger chisels and have become somewhat more 'brusque' in proceeding as compared to former times, I also attain my goal very rapidly.

"Even if one uses the saw, the chisel is eventually still required as one does not usually saw down to the dura. Though the surgeon may perform it as he wants, the practicing physician, who must however also be able to perform such an operation, has to be satisfied in general with the chisel. He should train with this instrument, which is much easier to handle than the saw, and after all is much less maneuverable. I have never seen any of the 'much feared' harmful effects of hammer-blows following a large number of chisel craniotomies, although I have carefully looked out for them. In a severe form, they seem to be met with most rarely. One should not fear such complications and they should certainly not constitute a contraindication for the use of the chisel."

Wagner's Osteoplastic Flap in the Literature

Wagner never depicted his flap, but the French pioneer neurosurgeon Antony Chipault did so (Fig 4) in his magnum opus *Chirurgie Opératoire du Système Nerveux*, which appeared in 1894. In his *Neurosurgery—An Historical Sketch*, Gilbert Horrax also illustrated Wagner's osteoplastic flap using the drawing from Chipault.

In 1930, Lambert Rogers in his most elaborate work, *History of Craniotomy*, gave an account of the methods that had been practiced and the instruments used for opening the human skull during life. Rogers pointed out that "One of the greatest advances in the method of opening the skull for surgical exploration of the brain

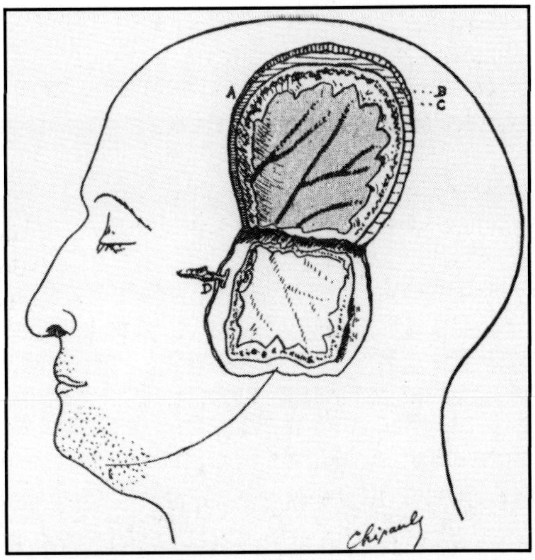

***Figure 4:** Wagner's osteoplastic flap as depicted by Antony Chipault. (From:* Chirurgie Opératoire du Système Nerveux. *Paris: Rueff et Cie; 1894:177.)*

and its investing membranes was that made in 1889 by Wilhelm Wagner of Königshütte. Osteoplastic craniotomy has now come to be known as Wagner's operation."

A Major French Contribution that Came too Late for Wagner

Wagner did not live to learn about the next major milestone in the history of cranial surgery: the solution to the problem of trephining without risks of producing intracranial damage presented by Count Thierry de Martel in 1908. Martel was already inquisitive as a boy and enjoyed taking mechanical things apart to learn how they operated. Frequently he dissected the fowl being prepared in the kitchen and he bought a skeleton, which he displayed as an amiable companion.

Martel, a descendant of the Mirabeau family, which played an outstanding role in the French Revolution, was an aristocrat who was fully conscious of his ancestry. He was primarily enrolled in a school for the training of engineers and was then trained by several French master surgeons. He became especially interested in neurosurgical instrumentation and at the age of 33, he published his milestone article describing two new neurosurgical instruments, both of which today, 90 years later, are in daily use by many thousands of neurosurgeons all over the world! In his presentation, Martel described the motor-driven trephine equipped with an automatic disengaging gear that stops the trephine as soon as it has penetrated the skull and the metal guide for the introduction of the Gigli saw between separate burr holes.

When in Paris, Martel presented his new automatic trephine, it was received with derision. He then performed a demonstration using a dried skull and placing a balloon on the inside in imitation of the dura mater. Thereafter, he drilled a hole in the skull with his automatic trephine without puncturing the balloon and commented: "Well as you can see, this trephine can be operated by an imbecile" ("et bien comme vous voyez, Messieurs, ce tréphan peut manié même par un imbécile").

By the late 1930s Martel's trephine and Wagner's osteoplastic flap were routinely used procedures in Scandinavia, France, Germany, and central Europe. Yet American neurosurgeons were especially reluctant to accept Martel's electric drill. In Boston in 1948, its use was rejected even at such a prominent place as the Massachusetts General Hospital. The burr holes were there done manually (and laboriously!) with Hudson drills. It was said that electric drills were not in use because Harvey Cushing once had stated that he had experienced that such drills caused too much vibration transmitted to the brain.

A sad end came to the great French pioneer Martel, who had lost his only son in World War I. In 1938, at the Annual Congress of the Deutsche Gesellschaft für Chirurgie, he gave an impassioned speech about the necessity of continued friendship between French and German surgeons, a speech that was followed by thunderous applause. As Hitler's troups occupied Paris this French neurosurgery pioneer committed suicide.

Conclusive Remark

All brain surgeons of today and their patients owe a respect to the remarkable pioneers who formed the basis of raising cranial flaps to explore diseases inside the cranial vault.

This quartet of pioneers came from four European cities in different countries: Wilhelm Wagner from Königshütte, Leonardo Gigli from Florence, Alfred Karol Obalinski from Cracow, and Thierry de Martel from Paris.

Selected References

1. Anonymous. Nekrolog. Wilhelm Wagner. *Die Medicinische Woche.* 1900;2:325-326.

2. Arendt (Kattowitz). Trepansäge. Bericht über die Verhandlungen der Deutschen Gesellschaft für Chirurgie, XXII Kongress 12/4-15/4 1893. *Beilage zum Centralblatt für Chirurgie.* 1893;30:21.

3. Bakay L. Ernst von Bergmann and the Cushing reflex. In: Bakay L. ed. *Neurosurgeons of the Past.* Springfield, Ill: Charles C Thomas Publisher; 1987:73-83.

4. Brock M. The small frontolateral approach for microsurgical treatment of intracranial aneurysms. *Neurochirurgie.* 1978;21:185-191.

5. Buchfelder M, Ljunggren B. Wilhelm Wagner (1848-1900) Part 1: A forgotten pioneer. *Surg Neurol.* 1988;30:423-427.

6. Buchfelder M, Ljunggren B. Wilhelm Wagner (1848-1900) Part 2: The osteoplastic flap. *Surg Neurol.* 1988;30:428-433.

7. Chipault A. *Chirurgie Opératoire du Système Nerveux.* Paris, France: Rueff et Cie; 1894.

8. de Martel T. Un point de technique opératoire dans la craniectomie. *Presse Med.* 1908;16:641-643.

9. Gigli L. Über ein neues Instrument zum Durchtrennen der Knochen, die Drahtsäge. *Zentralbl Chir.* 1894;21:409-411.

10. Gigli L. Zur praktischen Verwertung der Drahtsäge. *Zentralbl Chir.* 1897;24:785-788.

11. Gigli L. Zur Technik der temporären Schädelresektion mit meiner Drahtsäge. *Zentralbl Chir.* 1898;25:425-428.

12. Horrax G. Neurosurgery—An Historical Sketch. Springfield, Ill: Charles C Thomas Publisher; 1952:63.

13. Knötel P. Professor Dr. Wilhelm Wagner. Geheimer Sanitätsrat. Ein Gedenkblatt zur Enthüllung seines Denkmals in Königshütte. *Oberschlesien.* 1908;7:106-111.

14. Obalinski A. Zur Technik der Schädeltrepanation. *Zentralbl Chir.* 1897;24:857-859.

15. Pecker J. Thierry de Martel 1875-1940. *Surg Neurol.* 1980;13:401-403.

16. Rogers L. The history of craniotomy—an account of the methods which have been practiced and the instruments used for opening the human skull during life. *Annals of Medical History.* 1930;2:495-514.

17. Stenzel (Küstrin). Temporäre Schädelresektion. Bericht über die Verhandlungen der Deutschen Gesellschaft für Chirurgie, XXII Kongress 12/4-15/4 1893. *Zentralbl Chir.* 1893;30:27.

Neurosurgery in the 1700s

Olof af Acrel (1717-1806), the father of Swedish surgery (Fig 5), was surgeon-in-chief at the Royal Serafimer Hospital in Stockholm for an unprecedented period of 54 years in the 18th century. His work, "An Exhaustive Elucidation of the Properties of Fresh Wounds . . .," published in 1745, was the first scientific surgical study to appear in Sweden. His second work, "Surgical Events Observed at the Royal Hospital . . .," first published in 1759 (enlarged edition published in 1775), also was to become a milestone in Nordic surgery; Acrel compiled a description of surgical procedures of that time together with reports on several uncommon cases that he had encountered.

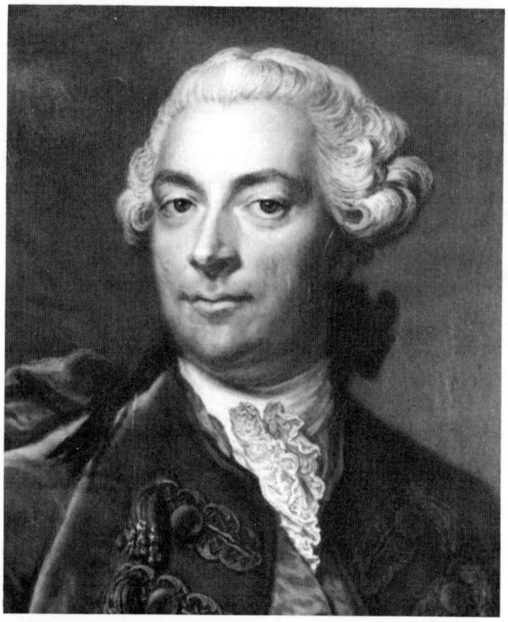

Figure 5: *Olof af Acrel (1717-1806)—the father of Swedish surgery (and neurosurgery).*

One such case report, in the 1775 edition, gives a thorough account of a nobleman 30 years old who had experienced a blow to his head and consequently for about a year had suffered from an increasing rather firm swelling of the cranium to the left of his crown. The nobleman had lost considerable weight and was remarkably pale, showing a slow but full pulse when Acrel finally was consulted. The patient was afflicted by an almost unbearable headache and insisted that Acrel should attempt a removal of the growth even if this might lead to his death.

Acrel was aware of one report concerning a similar case that had been published in 1743: a 34-year-old Prussian soldier, who was "also a gallant warrior in the Army of Venus," on whom the German pioneer in surgery, Lorenz Heister of Helmstedt, had operated, the case being presented in detail in a thesis by Dr. J.P. Kaufmann. With his own nonexistent experience of such cases, Acrel felt most dubious concerning an operative attempt but "was persuaded by several sensible men to have a try at resecting the tumor."

As he operated, Acrel found that the tumor growth, which was rather soft inside, had eroded the skull bone in the left frontoparietal region leaving a defect with irregular edges (Fig 6). The tumor was found to continue into the substance of the brain in the fore and middle lobes and to reach into the depth of the brain hemisphere, "thus allowing the introduction of the full length of my finger," he explained. "There was much arterial as well as venous hemorrhage" and Acrel's greatest concern was to achieve control of the bleedings, in which he was successful by applying "gradual pressure and rinsing of the tumor cavity with spirits." It is remarkable that despite lack of any form of anesthesia and with Acrel having introduced his finger deep into the brain, his patient survived the operation for three days—after which the patient died in severe convulsions.

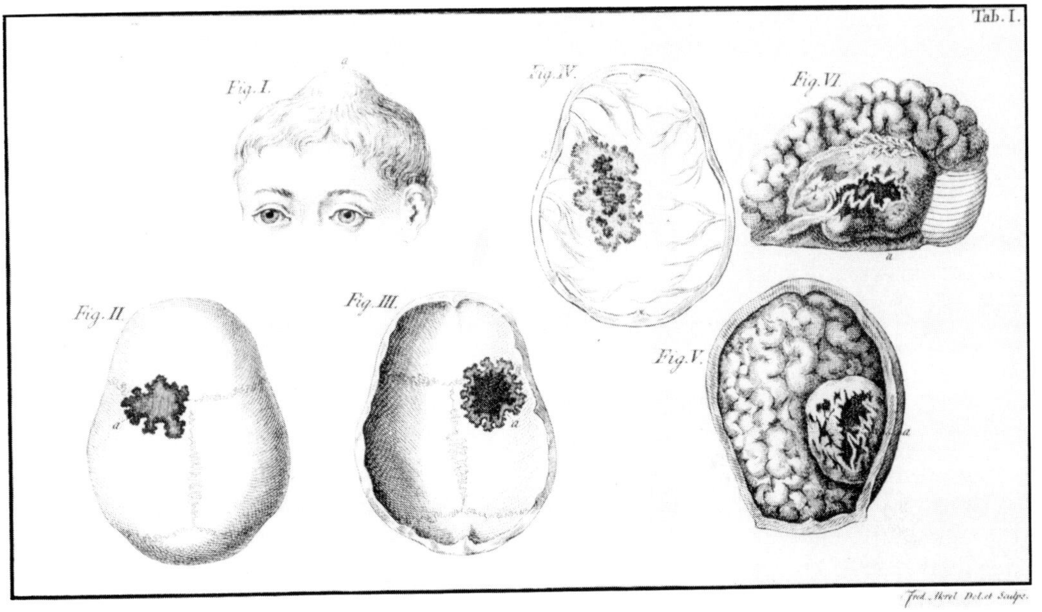

Figure 6: *Acrel's case of a cancerous tumor of the skull and brain, operated on in 1768.*

When Acrel published his case report, he was aware of a second case from the literature reported in 1772. This was a British fellow who served in the honorable Colonel Stewart's regiment in Dutch service and who was sent to Donald Monro (of the distinguished Monro medical family) because of a tumor above the left eyebrow with evident caries of the bone below. This tumor had increased gradually in the space of a year until it was the size of a hen's egg. The appearance of the tumor had deterred the British surgeons from attempting an operation. The soldier had then become lethargic, stuporous, and then totally incontinent, shortly after which he died.

Lieutenant-Colonel Georg Carl von Döbeln was a great hero in the war between Russia and Sweden in the years 1808-1809, which resulted in the loss of Finland from the Swedish Kingdom to its powerful eastern neighbor. He had been hit right between the eyes by a Russian musket ball in a previous war in 1789 at the battle of Porrassalmi. Acrel was present in 1791 when an attempt was made to perform an operative débridement. The operation was performed in Count von Horn's private home in Stockholm and was later vividly described by von Döbeln who followed the surgery via a hand mirror. "Anesthesia" was provided in the form of 15 drops of opium orally and does not seem to have been very effective: upon removal of the periosteum the pain was such that von Döbeln "shouted loudly." Unfortunately, he was not permanently cured. In the subsequent years right up to his death in 1820, he periodically suffered from suppuration and sequestration of small bony fragments from the Lesion (von Döbeln always described it with a capital letter), which he hid behind a black sweat band padded with chamois leather.

His heroic performances against the Russian enemy at the Battle of Juutas (1808) despite an exacerbation of the Lesion were depicted in Ensign Ståhl's Songs by Johan Ludvig Runeberg:

> "I must get well—and, though I were abiding
> deep in the grave, I must get on my feet.
> You hear the Russian guns at Juutas; they're deciding

the chances of our army's safe retreat.
And thither I must go ere it be shaken.
Is General Adlercreutz to be cut off and taken?
What will, then, be that army's fate at length?
No, write a line, from which—though it tomorrow
may make me tenfold worse—I yet may borrow,
for a few hours today, sufficient strength."

In summary, attempts were made already in the 1700s in Stockholm to remove visible brain tumors as well as to treat by surgery the complications arising after head injury.

Subarachnoid Hemorrhage with Catastrophic Consequences

When in the first week of May 1810 the Assembly of the Swedish Nation was brought to an end after year-long negotiations, the inhabitants of the kingdom finally breathed freely and entertained hopes for a future in peace after the hard times of the wars with Russia, upheavals, and domestic imbalance. Finland had been lost and incorporated with Tsarist Russia as a Grand Duchy, which meant that one-third of the original country and one-fourth of its inhabitants, nearly a million subjects, had been lost to Sweden forever. The king, Gustav Adolf IV, had been captured at the Royal Castle in Stockholm and forced to abdicate.

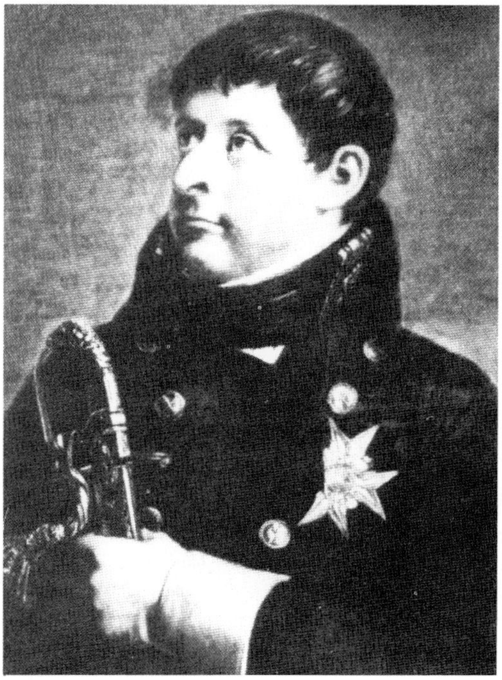

Figure 7: *Crown Prince Charles August of Sweden in early 1810. (From the Royal Palace of Sweden; reprinted with permission.)*

These dramatic events had been followed by the election of a founder of a new royal dynasty, the Danish count of Augustenborg, Christian August (Fig 7). Guidelines had been laid down for a new, more well-poised organization of the Swedish society. The 41-year-old prospective king had his name changed to the more royal sounding Charles August. As he was kind and friendly, he was popular in all classes of the Swedish society, the prospects for Sweden finally seemed favorable.

It was on forenoon Thursday, May 31, that a courier arrived in Stockholm with the disastrous news that during an inspection of two hussar regiments on Quidinge heath (some 100 kilometers north of Lund in southern Sweden) Charles August had suddenly fallen off his horse and died within an hour. Soon wild rumors circulated saying that Charles August had been poisoned. On June 20, during the funeral procession through the capital of Sweden, the agitation culminated. The completely innocent Marshal of the Realm, Count Axel von

Fersen, was forced to leave his carriage, his Golgotha-walk ending at the City Hall, where he was let into the guards' room. The mob, however, forced its way in and dragged out von Fersen to the courtyard where he was kicked and trampled to death (Fig 8). The murder of Count Axel von Fersen has been called the bottom mark of Swedish disgrace.

The protocol from the necropsy of Charles August, signed by three prominent professors from the University of Lund, arrived too late to prevent the terrible events at the funeral in the capital of Sweden. It ruled out any suspicion of poisoning and clearly showed that Charles August's death was occasioned by a spontaneous subarachnoid hemorrhage. And so it came that a subarachnoid hemorrhage led to a lynching that took place in broad daylight in the center of Stockholm.

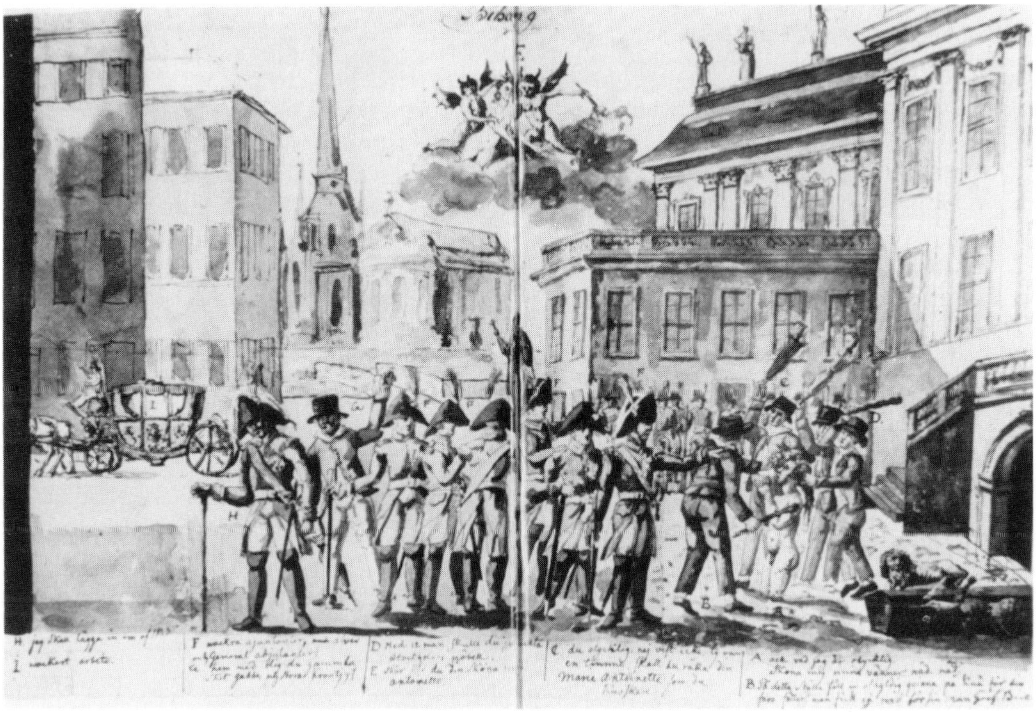

Figure 8: *Count Axel von Fersen begging for his life immediately before being beaten to death in central Stockholm. (From an engraving.)*

That the ruptured intracranial aneurysm, which with all certainty had caused the hemorrhage, was not discovered is not to be wondered at. The first clear report of it was not published until three years later by John Blackall, doctor of medicine at Oxford University. He then reported a similar case: a young previously healthy woman who had been struck by a cerebral apoplexia. Dr. Blackall described in detail the dramatic clinical course, which he observed carefully. And at the subsequent postmortem, he succeeded in tracing the meningeal hemorrhage to a ruptured aneurysm of the size of a horsebean at the top of the basilar artery. After the sudden and unexpected death of Charles August, in order to link Sweden closer to the French empire, a brother-in-law to Napoleon's brother, Marshal Jean Baptiste Bernadotte, count of Pontecorvo, was appointed to the Swedish throne (Fig 9).

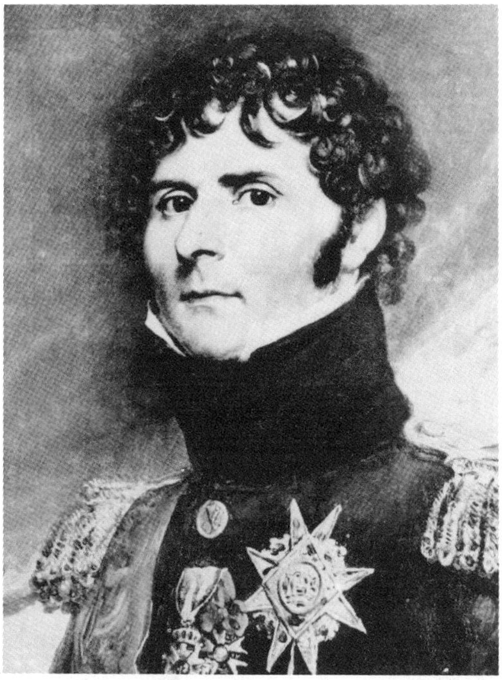

Figure 9: *King Charles XIV Johan of Sweden (Marshal Jean Baptiste Bernadotte). (From the Royal Palace of Sweden; reprinted with permission.)*

The present king of Sweden, Carl XVI Gustaf, is the seventh descendant in a direct line of this dynasty and thus with all probability owes his "royal patronage" to the rupture of an intracranial aneurysm some 179 years ago.

It was not until July 1932 that Egas Moniz and his assistant, the brain surgeon Almeida Lima, were able for the first time ever to visualize an intracranial aneurysm with their revolutionary new technique: cerebral angiography. The stage was then set for establishing the diagnosis of intracranial aneurysms and for consideration of their possible surgical treatment.

During the next decades little evidence arose favoring surgical treatment of these deadly lesions. The attitude was well reflected by the statement of Wardner Ayer in the mid 1930s: "Can surgery offer anything? The possibility of clipping off a small berry aneurysm on one of the communicating branches might be considered, but it would be a most formidable procedure and exceedingly dangerous, and the writer fears quite impracticable."

In 1931, Normann Dott of Edinburgh decided to operate on a formerly healthy active man who had experienced three subarachnoid hemorrhages within 14 days. After the last bleed, the patient had collapsed for some hours, but had again recovered apart from some degree of aphasia and an oculomotor nerve palsy. At the operation on April 22, two days after the last hemorrhage, "a formidable arterial hemorrhage filled the wound," said Dott, who "after following the right internal carotid artery to its bifurcation, removed a tenacious clot." With the aid of a suction apparatus, however, he was able to control the bleed while a colleague obtained fresh muscle from the patient's leg. Dott could see the spurting hemorrhage and was then able to "prepare a thick collar of muscle embedding the ruptured aneurysm and adjacent arterial trunks." The patient recovered so well that two years later he was fully able to indulge in shooting and mountaineering!

Dott maintained that Robert Louis Stevenson died of a subarachnoid hemorrhage from a ruptured aneurysm originating from the anterior communicating artery. The clinical symptoms, the type of intolerant headaches Stevenson had, and the type of akinetic mute state in which he was found prior to his death are highly suspicious in favor of Dott's opinion. This was a tragic end of a great man who himself had declared: "That man is a success who has lived well, laughed often and loved much; who has gained the respect of intelligent men and the love of children; who has filled his niche and accomplished his task; who leaves the world better than he found it, whether by an improved poppy, a perfect poem, or a rescued soul; who never lacked appreciation of earth's beauty or failed to express it; who looked for the best in others and gave the best he had."

In 1941, Professor Soma Weiss at the Peter Bent Brigham Hospital suffered a subarachnoid hemorrhage and himself diagnosed the bleed to be of aneurysmal origin—reported to be a ruptured middle cerebral artery aneurysm. None of the consulted neurosurgeons of the day felt that there was a surgical approach to the lesion. The death of Soma Weiss, with all probability caused by a new bleed, was a great loss to medicine and to mankind. He died of a lesion that today is easily recognized and in victims who "recover" after the first hemorrhage can be successfully treated with surgery.

Surgery of Traumatic Head Injury in the Early 1800s

Carl Daniel von Haartman, 1791-1877 (Fig 10), had visited Sir Astley Cooper in London in 1815-1816. He was appointed surgeon at the hospital of Turku (founded in 1756) in 1817. Turku was at this time the capital of Finland. The same year von Haartman performed a trepanation on a peasant who had a depressed skull fracture and severe brain injury. The bone fragments were partially removed and the patient recovered. Also, von Haartman described operations for dural sarcoma, spina bifida, and nasopharyngeal meningocele.

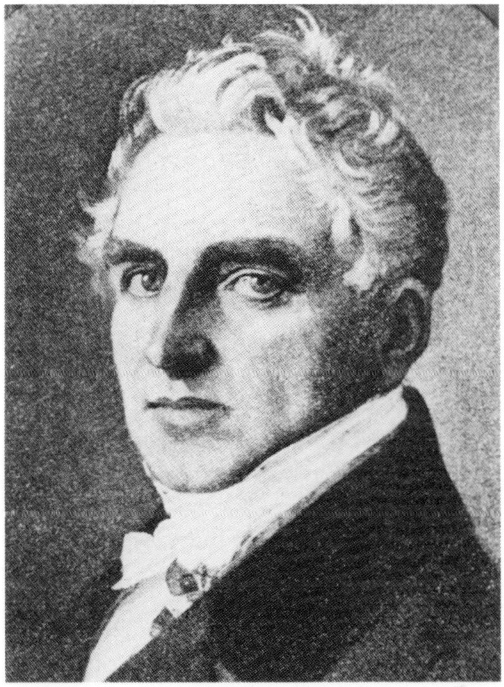

Figure 10: *Carl Daniel von Haartman (1791-1877).*

Arterial Ligation for Carotid-Cavernous Fistulas in the 1800s

Christopher Withusen (1778-1853) was surgeon-in-chief at the Royal Frederiks Hospital in Copenhagen. He had, like von Haartman, in 1816 visited Sir Astley Cooper in London. Withusen's younger colleague Gundelach Möller (1797-1845) in 1824 was awarded the gold medal of Copenhagen University for a historical review entitled "Exponere Historiam Ligaturae Arteriarum."

Both men were knowledgeable on a severe case that they had to handle. The patient was a four-year-old child with a congenital pulsating orbital growth. The decision was made to ligate the right common carotid artery and this was done on September 13, 1831. The pulsations disappeared but the patient developed a left hemiparesis; three months after surgery the pulsations appeared again. When in January 1832 the neurological deficits were dissolved, Gundelach Möller performed a ligation of the left common carotid artery as well. Following this procedure, performed without any anesthesia, the pulsations again disappeared. Eleven years later the patient died of smallpox and at the subsequent autopsy an encephalocele was found.

In 1864, Christopher Withusen's son David Withusen (1822-1874) ligated the right common carotid artery in a 44-year-old woman from Sweden who for about one year had suffered from a pulsating exophthalmos with severe pain on the affected side, chemosis, and visual failure. This operation, which also was performed without anesthesia, resulted in a temporary cure. A year later, there was a recurrence and the patient died.

Edvard Bull and a Case of Aneurysm 111 Years Ago

In 1877, the doctor of medicine of the Royal Fredriks University in Kristiania (now the University of Oslo) Edvard Bull, 1845-1925 (Fig 11), published a case report that bears witness to his outstanding farsightedness and most thorough knowledge of cerebrovascular disease. Bull was Henrik Ibsen's physician. Bull begins his essay by noting that the diagnosis of cerebral tumors is a highly difficult task. He then goes on to tell of a patient who had suffered meningeal apoplexy from rupture of an intracranial aneurysm. Quoting Bull's case report:

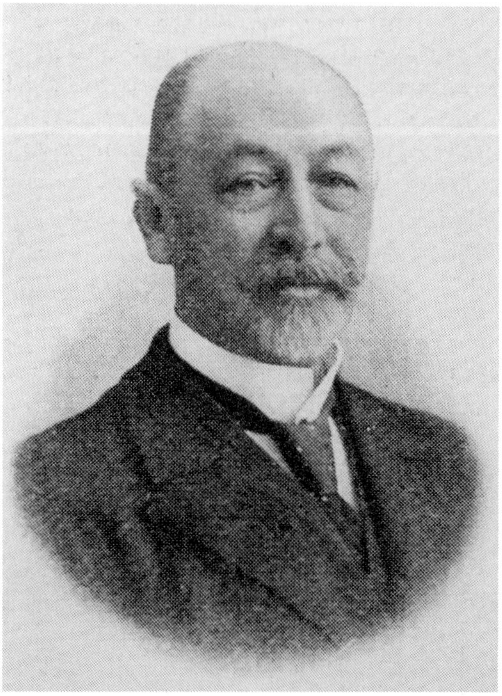

Figure 11: Edvard Bull (1845-1925).

> I was called to Oline Sofie K., aged 17, for the first time on the 27th of July 1877, because she was suffering from a headache; this had suddenly developed one of the days in the week now past, while she was sitting and straining at a troublesome exoneratio alvi: during this procedure, she sensed of a sudden that "something had gone off" inside her head above the right eye, and during her entire illness the headache remained confined to this part of the head. The pain showed a pronounced tendency to temporary remission. In addition, there was periodic vomiting, constipation, and slight fever. That was the history of the case.

At his examination of the sick girl on July 28, Bull diagnosed a meningeal apoplexy and a third nerve palsy. He treated the patient with cold compresses on the head and dispensed laxatives, potassium iodide mixtures, and morphine. No pronounced change took place during the following days, except that the girl's ptosis increased so that finally on August 1 she could not open her eyelid at all. At this time, her right pupil also was dilated and showed no reaction to light.

During the subsequent weeks, however, her general condition showed a steady improvement, she regained her appetite and began to feel generally better. Notwithstanding this, Bull apprised the parents that their daughter was in immediate danger of her life. He expressed his doubts as to her chances of recovering her health, realizing that she had suffered from rupture of an intracranial aneurysm exerting pressure on the right oculomotor nerve. On the basis of his experiences from similar cases he concluded that the presumed aneurysm could again rupture at any time with fatal consequences.

The catastrophe soon occurred as predicted by Bull. On August 30 his patient, having got up in the morning as usual, suddenly at 10:45 am lost consciousness and exhibited severe convulsions. "She was waving her arms violently about; her mouth was drawn over to the right; on my arrival 30 minutes later she was dead." At the autopsy of Oline Sofie K. a ruptured aneurysm originating from the right internal carotid artery at the takeoff of the posterior communicating artery and exerting pressure on the oculomotor nerve was found, which was exactly the lesion that Bull had diagnosed.

In his discussion of the case, Bull concludes that there is neither medical nor surgical therapy available in the treatment of ruptured intracranial aneurysms. However, he emphasized that carotid ligation might have been worth considering for the prevention of further bleedings. Bull's case description and the workings of his mind testify to his being at least 50 years ahead of his time.

Forty-three years were to pass before the young British physician Charles Symonds drew Harvey Cushing's attention to the fact that a patient who was due for surgery of a suspected brain tumor was probably in fact suffering from a ruptured intracranial aneurysm. Cushing received this supposition with scepticism; when he operated, he found that Symonds had been right and that there was in fact a subarachnoid hemorrhage. The patient died during the night after the operation, and Cushing immediately had Symonds devote himself to specialized studies of aneurysms of cerebral arteries and the consequences of their rupture. Three years later, Symonds published his findings; his work constituted a breakthrough for the diagnosis of subarachnoid hemorrhage in North America.

In 1928, on the initiative of the neurologist Fuller Albright in Baltimore, Walter Dandy ligated the carotid artery in a patient suffering from an aneurysm exerting pressure on the oculomotor nerve—that is to say, he performed the very operation that Edvard Bull had proposed half a century before. The value of Dandy's pioneering effort is in no way diminished by the fact that his patient died after surgery or that Edvard Bull's compatriot Vilhelm Magnus had already in the previous year succeeded in ligating the internal carotid artery in a 69-year-old man suffering from intractable trigeminal neuralgia.

Vilhelm Magnus suspected that his patient was suffering from a slowly growing brain tumor exerting pressure on the gasserian ganglion. As the patient's condition was unbearable, Magnus performed an operation to remove the trigeminus root. As the dura mater was detached from the base of the cranium, Magnus said that he "came on a tumor about the size of a chestnut with a smooth surface and glistening like mother of pearl, strictly limited and situated on the surface of the gasserian ganglion." During his further attempts at detaching the dura from the surface of the tumor, a hole was torn and the contents of the tumor poured out. About half of the content was emptied when there was "a great gush of blood, that could not be stopped by tamponade." Then, Magnus ligated the internal carotid artery and the bleeding stopped. Afterwards the trigeminus root was removed. This case was reported by Magnus in the Journal of the American Medical Association in May 1927 under the title "Aneurysm of the internal carotid artery; clinical notes, suggestions, and new instruments." Magnus there noted that "the patient stood the operation very well and had declared to Magnus that he could not have been given a better birthday gift, as he had completed his sixty-ninth year on the day of surgery" (Fig 12).

Vilhelm Magnus (1871-1929)—Pioneer Brain Surgeon

Vilhelm Magnus (Fig 13) received his medical training at Oslo University. His great interest in further study led him to Paris in 1898 where he applied himself to neurology and histology. He continued to Frankfurt am Main, studying neuroanatomy and neuropathology under Carl Weigert and Ludwig Edinger at the famous Senckenberg Institute (Fig 14).

In Breslau, he was initiated into experimental embryology at the Institute of Professor Born, and he was later able to furnish scientific proof of Born's hypothesis of an active

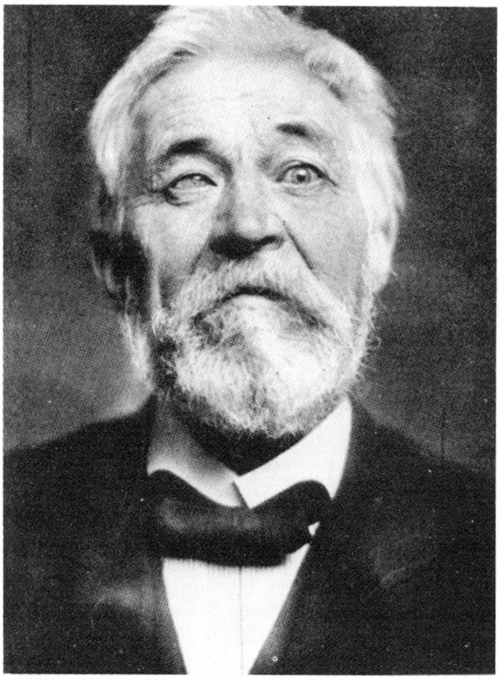

Figure 12: *Vilhelm Magnus' patient with aneurysm of internal carotid artery.*

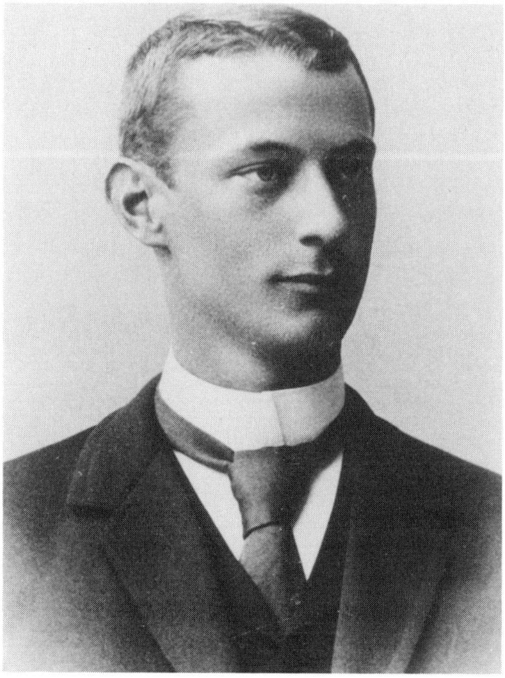

Figure 13: *Vilhelm Magnus (1871-1929).*

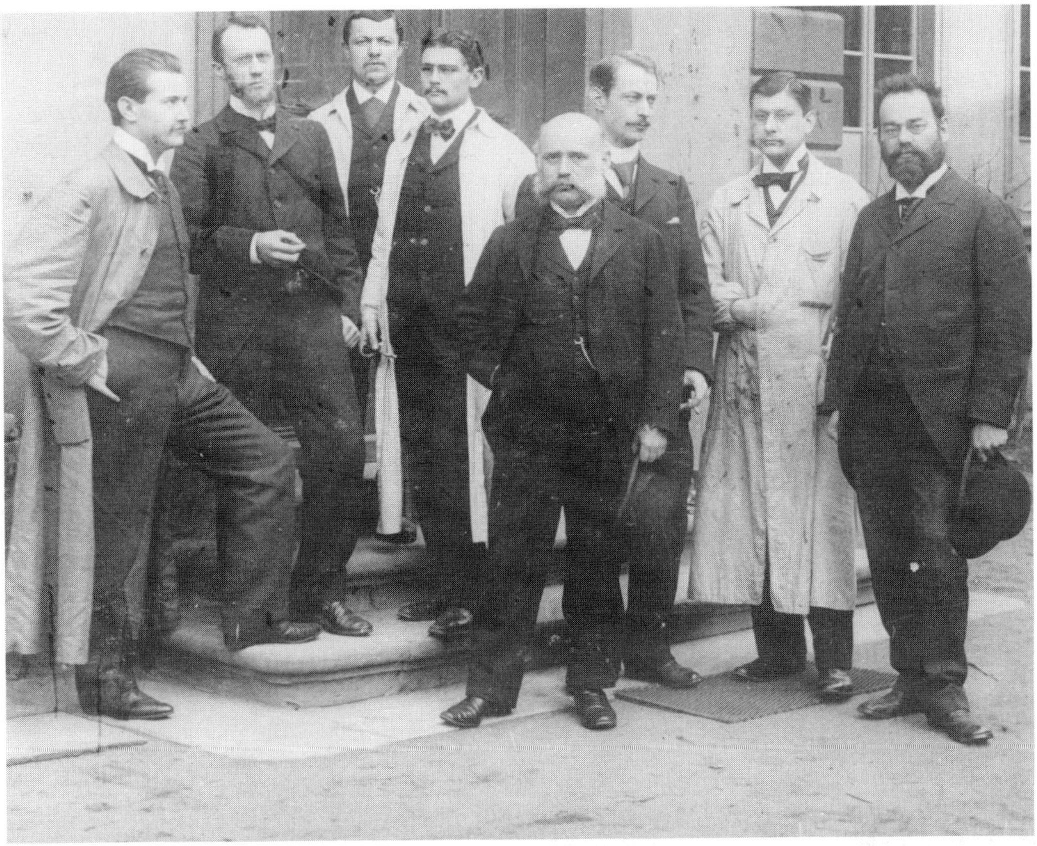

Figure 14: At the Senckenberg Institute—Vilhelm Magnus standing to the right behind Carl Weigert.

secretion from the corpus luteum. Thus, in 1901, Vilhelm Magnus was the first person in the world to demonstrate the occurrence of the substance that many years later was given the designation progesterone (the word hormone was not yet in existence; it was used for the first time in 1905 by Starling at Hardy's suggestion).

After Breslau, Magnus went to London to train as a brain surgeon under Victor Horsley, the first neurosurgeon who fully realized the value of establishing close collaboration with colleagues within neurology, physiology, and pathology. From his stay with Horsley in 1904 Magnus reported:

> "In London there is a unique opportunity—as probably nowhere else—to observe a series of brain and spinal cord operations during a relatively short period. Horsley has practically a monopoly, and with good reason because hardly anyone has been so well qualified to be a pioneer. His basis in physiology acquired through many years' experiments on animal brains is combined with an unusual ability of observation and swift and meticulous action. His results are brilliant, and he may for instance perform an explorative laminectomy on indications which for the less knowledgeable may seem doubtful.

"His technical skill in operations on the central nervous system may be illustrated by the successful removal of a pituitary tumor in a patient with acromegaly with a favorable outcome. His technique is the simplest possible, as it must be under the conditions prevailing for London surgeons. It is not becoming for a doctor to run a private clinic in England, and thus they must operate in nursing homes. Some of the ones I visited had no operating theater, and Horsley operated in the bedroom where the thick carpet was not removed. In others, a small operating room was arranged in a former garden cottage. He also performed operations in the patients' homes. Under such circumstances, the British surgeon must learn to use the least complicated equipment and to work under what we would call primitive conditions. For the same reasons antisepsis prevailed. Sublimate in strong alcoholic solutions was virtually considered a magic water, a few seconds' rinsing of the hands in this fluid being regarded sufficient. But on the basis of bad experience, the British surgeon has seen the danger of a superficial antisepsis and has learned to operate with instruments.

"The most surprising thing in London was to observe how little the surgeons touched the wound with their fingers. Horsley for instance performed extirpations of the gasserian ganglion without touching the field with his fingers. The use of rubber gloves was common. Another surprising observation was the untrained assistants. Residents are not found in the London hospitals, only house surgeons, young newly graduated physicians in a few places, but most often students, and they change every three to four months."

In an obituary published after Sir Victor Horsley's premature death in Mesopotamia in 1916, Magnus concluded the following:

"Undoubtedly, Sir Victor Alexander Horsley—the creator of neurosurgery—became considered as one of the great leaders of British medicine, although his literary production in terms of the number of pages was not that impressive. But in England, people judge by other criteria than the mere number of published pages. Already as a very young doctor he became a pioneer in everything he undertook. At age 27, he was the first to show that the thyroid gland has an internal secretion, and he proposed that myxedema patients should be treated with thyroid gland transplants. Two years later, he gained a world reputation after a successful removal of a cerebral tumor, and in the following year he removed a spinal tumor. At the National Hospital, he had to perform brain tumor surgery in a small corner of a ward only demarcated by movable screens, and later in an auditorium not equipped for surgical use. It was only during his final years that he was given a modest operating theater.

"His technical skill as a neurosurgeon was phenomenal and may be exemplified by the fact that so far no one else had succeeded in the extirpation of pituitary tumors via the temporal approach. Horsley had performed this operation in 10 patients without mortality several years before any other surgeon even thought of surgery for such lesions.

"In his small miserable cave of a laboratory at University College—dirty, cramped, and very poorly equipped—Horsley was in his right element. There he regularly performed experiments on certain afternoons regardless of the amount of clinical practice. His immense diligence resulted in a universal knowledge of experimental physiology, neurology, anatomy, pathology, surgery, archeology, history, and politics. He stood head and shoulders above all the other consultants and for that reason was called the consultant of consultants.

"Horsley was one of those giants who materialize at long intervals. Courageous, chivalrous, and without concern about his own person, glowing with the holy fire of indignation when detecting something he considered wrong, he hit as hard as was to be expected from a man as strong as him. This was sometimes interpreted as belligerence and intolerance although it was really a manifestation only of a most straightforward and self-sacrificing character. His sense of justice and admiration for the good and right made him a born reformer and he consequently immediately volunteered for war service in the ill-fated Mesopotamian campaign when he learned of the miserable conditions there.

"It may be claimed that it was a pity that Horsley did not publish his neurosurgical results in a monograph. He often mentioned it himself—with a humorous glint in his penetrating grey eyes. However, his interests were so manifold and his working time so extremely occupied that it would have been a waste of time."

In 1903, Vilhelm Magnus performed his first two-stage operation on a deep-seated tumor in the left cerebral hemisphere of a 47-year-old man. The patient had presented epileptic fits accompanied by right-sided paralysis and speech impediments. Eighteen years later Magnus published his "Bidrag til hjernechirurgiens klinikk og resultate" ("On clinical practice and results in brain surgery") in the Norwegian medical periodical *Norsk Magazin for Laegevidenskaben.* He based his study on experience from 112 patients on whom he had operated for brain tumors. The surgical mortality was 8 percent, a phenomenal result for the time. His study also covered patients with epilepsy, trigeminal neuralgia, and some other neurosurgical diseases.

The most remarkable fact in all is that Magnus held no post at the university. He performed all his operations at small private hospitals, and without the aid of a single trained assistant until the last years, when he received help from a colleague named Knudtzon.

If his unprecedented results failed to gain international recognition, this must most probably be ascribed to the fact that, with the exception of two articles, he published his total of 70 scholarly works only in Norwegian in spite of his fluency in the English and French languages.

In 1913, Magnus started doing palliative craniectomies followed by radiotherapy in pituitary tumors. His diagnoses were based on radiographic investigations of the sellar region, ophthalmoscopy, and visual tests including repeated examinations of visual field defects. He published a series of studies on this subject in the years from 1916 to 1925, in which year he also presented his overall results of brain tumor surgery at the annual meeting of the Scandinavian Surgical Association in Copenhagen. He had by then operated on 189 patients with brain tumors, the surgical mortality being 7.7 percent for supratentorial tumors and 17.8 percent for posterior fossa tumors.

Magnus' Impressions of American Neurosurgery in the Year 1928

A year before his death, Vilhelm Magnus accompanied a patient to Boston and paid a five-week visit to Harvey Cushing's by then world-famous clinic at the Peter Bent Brigham Hospital in Boston. In a typewritten report Magnus gives his "Impressions of American Neurosurgery":

> "My visit is limited to five weeks in Boston. I consider it more worth while to stay just at one place for a little longer than to fritter away one or two days at each of several hospitals: one cannot study in depth on such a tour, cannot grow familiar with all those small technical refinements which are the distinguishing marks of any particular school. At present, Cushing is the undisputed leader in surgery of the nervous system because he, more than any other, developed a school gathering about him pupils whom he sets to work. From him and his pupils, there come a quantity of publications every year.
>
> "He himself is eager to hear the latest findings, continually testing new methods of both examination and operation. Thus in his department, over the past two years or so, use has been made of a technique with diathermy scalpels, this being a great advance for the extirpation of endotheliomas or meningiomas, the bloodiest of all these operations. Diathermy has been employed twice or more for the successful extirpation of such benign tumors which with an ordinary technique would have been hazardous due to the profuse bleeding from the diploë and dura mater. This device was said to be the only one that had been made outside the laboratory, but one that would soon be on the market—doubtless at a price to make us Europeans faint.
>
> "The Peter Bent Brigham Hospital is disorderly and in parts unhygienic, because there is not the same washing and scrubbing as we are used to from our hospitals, brooms being used first on all floors before they are swabbed, probably because they are afraid that the thick linoleum—battleship linoleum—which is used will rot if it is washed too much. There are employed nurses without number with their helpers, and helpers in the form of lady typists and stenographers, secretaries and undersecretaries, keepers of the lists and more. . . . The operations rendered an impression of great cleanliness. If a bloody swab fell on the floor, it was plucked up on the instant—clearly, the staff were highly anxious to preserve the immaculate condition of their white tiled floor!
>
> "The extirpation of brain tumors proceeded with the greatest caution and with the use of a number of small technical tricks. Cushing was full of expedients for arresting bleeding: it was a pleasure to see how free from blood his operations were, and the care he took to stem even the slightest hemorrhage.

"He said that he considered the operations for tumors of the eighth cranial nerve to be the most exacting ones he knew, and he had harsh judgment to pronounce on those surgeons who without the requisite experience undertook these operations, which in the hands of an inexperienced surgeon were desperate remedies indeed. He was also sharp in his condemnation of those surgeons who set about brain operations after only having witnessed one or two of them before. I have never known a surgeon who took such pains with every single patient as Cushing did. The mainspring of his work was his boundless anxiety about his statistics—that the mortality should not exceed 10 percent."

When Herbert Olivecrona Started

In Sweden, brain surgery is often, and with every right, connected with the name of Herbert Olivecrona (1891-1981)—the trailblazer and the foreground figure within this modern surgical speciality. At the same time as Harvey Cushing was serving at field hospitals on the Western Front, the young Olivecrona's (Fig 15) inquiring mind was beginning to learn about surgical treatment of bullet and shrapnel wounds of the head and spine at German military hospitals.

Another Swedish surgeon who was taking the opportunity to gain experience of army medical services was Einar Key (1872-1954), who toured a large number of battlefields and several prison camps on the German side and who was even allowed to travel on a hospital train fetching casualties on the Western Front.

In 1922, at the age of 31 years and as junior surgeon at the surgical department of the Serafimer Hospital in Stockholm, Olivecrona operated on his first brain case. The patient, suffering from a metastasis that Olivecrona did not succeed in localizing, survived surgery but developed a brain herniation and died.

His second case, a patient with an acoustic nerve tumor, was somewhat more successful. One difficulty was to supply the patient, lying face down as required for the exploration, with sufficient quantities of ether for inhalation. The result was that during the operation the patient was at times more or less conscious. The anesthetist, or "dropper" as was the designation at that time, became so affected by the ether vapors under the operating table that he was put out and had to be dragged forth in an anesthetized condition. The patient survived for 18 days, which caused quite a sensation.

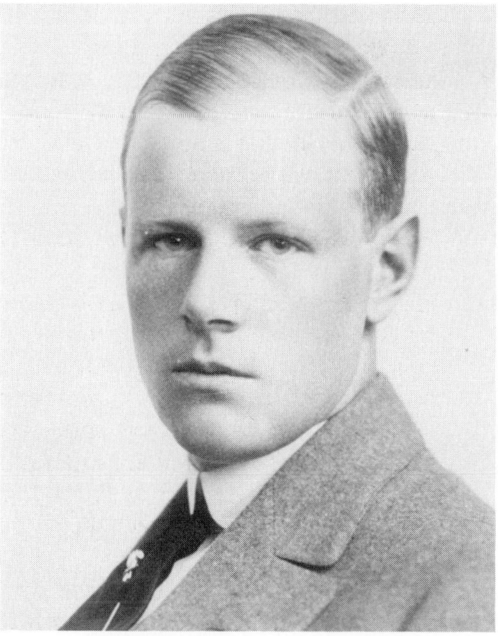

Figure 15: *Herbert Olivecrona at the age of 26 (1917).*

Nordic Pioneering Spirit

The end of the 18th and beginning of the 19th century was an era of significant scientific progress and important discoveries. It is probably no coincidence that some of the outstanding pioneers of these achievements were acquainted with each other. Thus Vilhelm Magnus studied medicine with the Norwegian explorer Roald Amundsen (1872-1928), who abandoned medicine for arctic ventures. And the Swedish explorer of Central Asia, Sven Hedin (1865-1952), established a close relationship with Einar Key and Harvey Cushing.

Cushing appears to have held the surgery being carried out in Scandinavia during the opening decades of this century in high esteem. In the late summer of 1929, he visited Sweden, and in October he once again met Sven Hedin and Einar Key in Boston. In December of the same year he wrote to Key, "I can't tell you how delighted I am with that plaque of your father (Fig 16). I shall keep it in my library as near to the volumes of his works as it can possibly go and I will feel that his scientific spirit hovers over my quarters."

The volumes to which Cushing was alluding were the 1875 monograph *Anatomie des Nervensystems und des Bindegewebes* published by Gustaf Retzius and Einar's father, Axel Key (see Fig 19, in Chapter 3). In his famous 1925 Cameron lecture in Edinburgh, Cushing had said of this work that "we need not forget that it is precisely 50 years since Key and Retzius published their monumental contribution to our knowledge of the intracranial spaces" (Fig 17).

The epithet "monumental" might have had a double meaning, for the size of this work is overwhelming—two folios with a total weight of about 20 pounds.

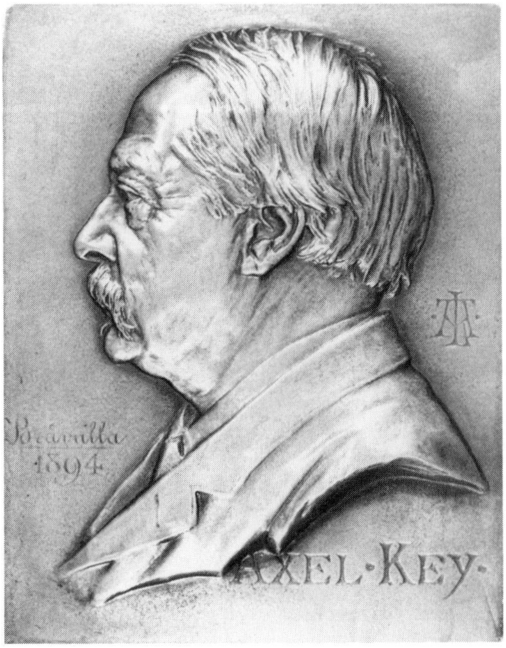

Figure 16: *Plaque of Axel Key.*

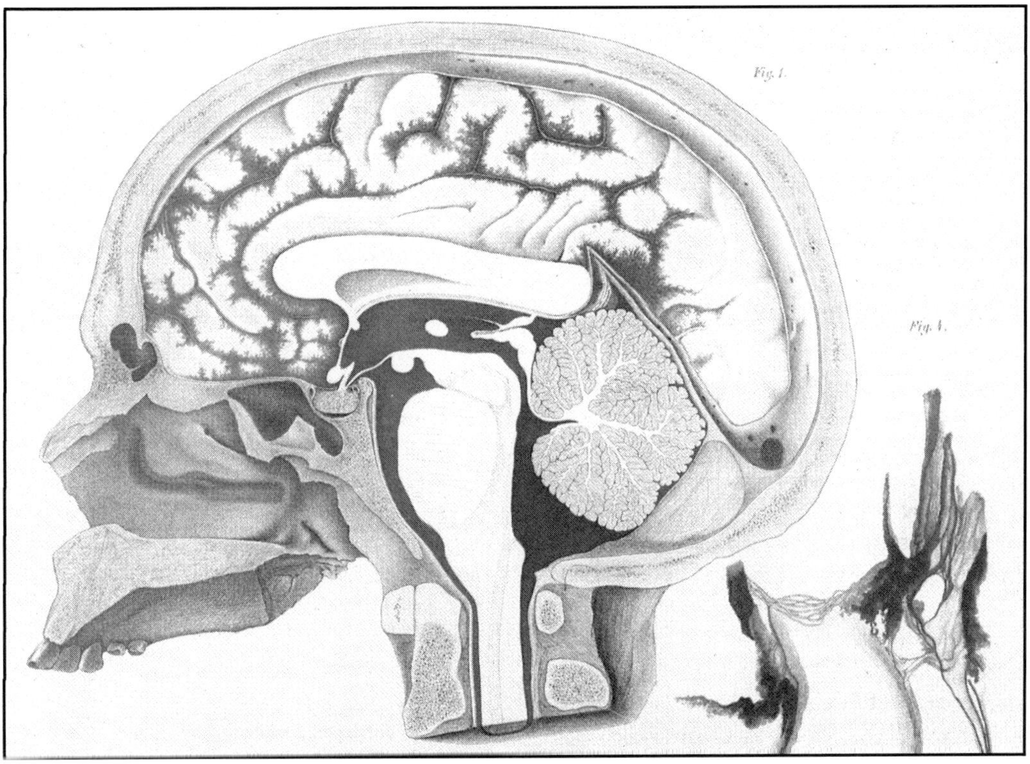

Figure 17: *Drawing from 1875 work by Key and Retzius.*

Selected References

1. af Acrel O. An exhaustive elucidation of the properties of fresh wounds. Stockholm, Sweden: H. Fougt; 1745.

2. af Acrel O. Cranii cerebrique fungus cancrosus—observations from the year 1768. In: *Surgical Events.* Stockholm, Sweden: H. Fougt; 1775:25-30.

3. Albright F. The syndrome produced by aneurysm at or near the junction of the internal carotid artery and the circle of Willis. *Johns Hopkins Hosp Bull.* 1929;44:215-245.

4. Amneus AJ. Concerning the manner of death of crown prince Charles August (Karl August) and the medico-legal main points in the trial against his physician Rossi [in Swedish]. *Upsala University Year-Book.* Upsala, Sweden: Upsala University; 1865:1-89.

5. Ask-Upmark E, Ingvar D. A follow-up examination of 138 cases of subarachnoid haemorrhage. *Acta Med Scand.* 1950;88:15-31.

6. Ayer WD. So-called spontaneous subarachnoid haemorrhage. A resumé with its medicolegal consideration. *Am J Surg.* 1934;26:143-151.

7. Blackall J. Observations on the nature and cure of dropsies. 5th ed. London, England: Longman & Co; 1813:132-135.

8. Bull E. Akut Hjerneaneurisma—Okulomotoriusparalyse—meningealapoplexi. *Norsk Magazin Laegevidenskaben.* 1877;7:890-895.

9. Cushing H. Contributions to the study of intracranial aneurysms. *Guys Hosp Rec.* 1923;73:159-163.

10. Cushing H. Correspondence to Einar Key. Stockholm, Sweden: Karolinska Institute Library; 1929.

11. Dott NM. Intracranial aneurysms: cerebral arterio-radiography; surgical treatment. *Edin Med J.* 1933;40:219-240.

12. Gejrot T. Om Döbeln och hans Blessur. *Swed Med J.* 1966;63:2565-2571.

13. Hellström J. Einar Key's contributions to surgery. *Acta Chir Scand.* 1954;108:85-93.

14. Kaufmann JP. Dissertatio de tumore capitis fungoso post cariem cranii exorto. In: Haller A, ed. *Disputationes Chirurgicae Selectae.* Lausanne, Switzerland; 1775:45-62.

15. Key A, Retzius G. *Studien in der Anatomie des Nervensystems und des Bindegewebes.* 1st & 2nd vols. Stockholm, Sweden: Norstedts; 1875.

16. Klossner AR. *Provincial Hospital of Turku* 1756-1856 [in Finnish]. Turku, Finland: University of Turku; 1956.

17. Lundberg N. The saga of the Monro-Kellie Doctrine. In: Ishii S, Brock M, eds. *Intracranial Pressure V.* Berlin, Germany: Springer Verlag; 1983:68-75.

18. Magnus V. Aneurysm of the internal carotid artery. *JAMA.* 1927;88:1712-1713.

19. Magnus V. Bidrag til hjernechirurgiens klinikk og resultater. *Norsk Magazin for Laegevidenskaben.* 1921;(suppl):1-138.

20. Magnus V. *Erfaringer fra 20-aars hjernekirurgii.* Lecture. Scandinavian Surgical Society Annual Meeting; Copenhagen; June 25-27, 1925. Oslo, Norway: Steenske Boktrykkeri (Johannes Björnstad). 1925:193-197.

21. Magnus V. Et tilfaelde av hypofysetumor behandlet med organoterapi. *Norsk Magazin for Laegevidenskaben.* 1916;77:1319-1326.

22. Magnus V. *Inntryk av amerikansk neurokirurgi.* Visit to Boston (Harvey Cushing). 1928. Typescript.

23. Magnus V. Operativ og Röntgen-behandling av hypofysetumores. *Forhandlinger i Medicinsk Selskab.* Oslo, Norway; 1923:92-94.

24. Magnus V. Ovariets betydning for svangerskabet med saerlig hensyn til corpus luteum. *Norsk Magazin for Laegevidenskaben.* 1901:1138-1145.

25. Magnus V. Rapport til Det Akademiske Kollegium, Det Kgl. In: Handwritten report to the Academy of Oslo University. Oslo, Norway: Fredriks Universitet; 1904.

26. Möller G. Underbinding af de primitive carotider foretagen på Det kgl. Frederik's Hospital. *Bibliotek for Laeger.* 1932;17:56-68.

27. Moniz E. Anévrysme intra-cranien de la carotide inferne droite rendu visible par l'artériographie cérébrale. *Rev Otoneuroophtalmol.* 1933;11:746-748.

28. Monro D. An account of some uncommon cases. *Medical Trans Lond.* 1772;2:353-358.

29. Olivecrona H. *Die Chirurgische Behandlung der Gehirntumoren.* Berlin, Germany: Springer Verlag; 1927.

30. Söderhjelm A. *Georg Carl von Döbeln.* Stockholm, Sweden; 1937.

31. Sögaard I. Tidlig neurokirurgi i Danmark. In: *Dansk Medicinsk Historisk Årbog.* Copenhagen, Denmark; 1986:153-165.

32. Symonds CP. Contributions to the clinical study of intracranial aneurysms. *Guys Hosp Rep.* 1923;72:139-158.

33. Törmä T. Perspectives in international neurosurgery: neurosurgery in Finland. *Neurosurgery.* 1981;9:479-481.

34. von Bonsdorff B, Palmgren E, trans. *The History of Medicine in Finland, 1882-1918.* Helsinki, Finland: Societas Scientarium Fennica; 1975.

Chapter 3

When Nobel First Told of His Testament—The Nobel Prize in Medicine

When Alfred Nobel met Axel Key (the rector of the Karolinska Institute) on the Riviera in April 1893, he revealed for the first time his plans to found an international prize in medicine. It was only a few weeks earlier that he had made out a will providing for the Karolinska Institute to reward outstanding discoveries within "the domain of physiology and medicine."

Key gave an account of his remarkable encounter with Nobel in a letter to his wife Selma in Stockholm. This letter gives a fascinating picture of the times and a unique portrait of the shy and retiring Nobel.

Who Was Axel Key?

Axel Key was born on October 25, 1832, at Johannisberg Manor near Jönköping in Småland, Sweden. His youth passed in private studies free from the compulsion to attend school. He himself considered that this liberal early education favorably disposed him to the great zest and enjoyment of work and activity that characterized the rest of his life. By the age of 16, he was a student and by 29 a professor.

Key's medical studies at the University of Lund coincided with the golden age of pathological anatomy in the middle years of the 19th century. In 1860-1861 he spent more than a year in Germany, studying histology under Max Schultze in Bonn and pathology and physiology under Rudolf Virchow in Berlin.

Soon after returning home, he publicly defended a dissertation on sensory nerve endings in the frog's tongue; and in the same year, he was appointed professor of pathological anatomy at the Karolinska Institute. He preferred not to wear the aura of a learned man, being too sociable and unauthoritarian for such a style. He understood, as few others have done, how to captivate the interest of his students. Even when well advanced in years, he would still participate in the social gatherings of his students. He was for many years the inspector of the Swedish Medical Society, later becoming an honorary member.

Study Trip Through Central Europe in 1872

In order to forge more numerous links with universities abroad, Axel Key embarked in the autumn of 1872 on a journey to central Europe and visited a large number of seats of learning. His impressions are preserved in letters to his wife, and they show great discernment in the assessment of those then practicing medical science.

He expressed his admiration for gifted and inventive men and for sound research, but also his indignation over scholars whose textbooks showed that they had taken over sections and "loaned" illustrations from his own works without citing the originator. One professor of pathology in Amsterdam inspired him with but little confidence: "He appeared to have laid aside his science as far as possible, seeking instead to cut broad strips out of the hides of the Amsterdamers, sharing with them the profits from the colonial trade. Notwithstanding, he was very friendly and attentive, giving a dinner etc.—and yet, as it seemed to me, with the quite apparent calculation not to expend upon a foreigner too much of the good things which he had been able with difficulty and labor to garner home. And I daresay that was just as well."

Low Scientific Ambitions in Belgium

Things were not much better in Brussels. Once again, Key found the scientific life of the place somewhat disheartening. He remarked, "It is all done only for show. The professors employ the position they hold merely in order to gain importance in the eyes of the public and to win a large clientele. Their teaching is a miserable affair, whose virtual sole aim is to give a brief résumé of what has been accomplished elsewhere. Yet not even this is within their compass, lacking acquaintance as they do with the progress of the science beyond their own borders. But what is worse, these dismal conditions do not obtain in Brussels alone, they are the measure for the whole of Belgium. Many were the professors I met who frankly declared with deep melancholy that Belgium in the realm of science had fallen so low that they could not conceive of its rescue."

In Leuven (Louvain), Key found that science stood at an even lower level than in Brussels, "and what is worse, it appears to lack the consciousness of its miserable state, being on the contrary full of Catholic unction and superstition."

There, he met a professor of surgery, "about whom I do not believe that surgical science has anything to relate, but who in the course of half an hour's conversation essayed to render credible to me that he was a man of great excellence whose repute had traveled far beyond the sea, so that people would make the voyage from America just to be rendered happy by his knife." A fetid smell in his hospital caused Key to inquire whether numbers of patients did not die of pyemia after their operations. The answer was that one surgical patient in four died of this complication and "the precautionary measures now being applied for the prevention of this disease were here entirely unknown." Key was shocked, noting that he would never have believed such ignorance possible at a university hospital.

Ingenious Instruments

Liège was altogether different. Here, Key met the aging Schwann and said, "one of the noblest persons of our science, who laid the cornerstones of all the knowledge which is under culture in the medical field with the aid of the microscope." He "surprised the old man in the middle of a physiological experiment, using the most ingenious instruments, which he had designed himself." Key found Schwann to be one of the most amiable personalities he had ever met, remarking that the dinner in the later part of the evening was the most pleasant and stimulating he had yet experienced.

Professors of the First Order

After his visit with Schwann, Key proceeded to Paris, where he expressed his disappointment at the laboratory appointed for the use of Ranvier and Claude Bernard, the latter "a professor of physiology of the first order."

Pressing on to the new German university in Strassburg, he called in on Recklinghausen and described him as "a superb scientist and a man of honor," who devoted to his Swedish guest "all the time at his disposal for two days, notwithstanding all the hustle and bustle at the beginning of the new term with its convocations and clamour." In

Heidelberg, Key met the physiologist Wilhelm Kühne, whom he characterized as one of the great German geniuses of medicine.

In Zürich he was struck by the large number of women, mostly Russians, who were studying medicine and said, "This was somewhat curious, but it has proved to work excellently, with neither annoyance nor conflict."

Low Scientific Standard in Italy

In Florence, Key said that he came across "quite a celebrity, his name is Pacini: a straightforward elderly Italian who was extremely eager to demonstrate new microscope designs which he had made but whom one could induce by no means to enter upon any other subjects." Key soon confirmed his suspicions that Pacini "had been neglecting his real field of study for quite some time, so that the knowledge of today was unfamiliar to him."

In Siena he made the acquaintance of several professors with very different personalities. The anatomist was "an old, befogged and extremely benevolent man, who weighed and reweighed 15 times upon the scales of his erstwhile intellection whether he should give me two dissertations or whether they might not by their insignificance reduce his stature. At length, seizing the pen, he inscribed each with a flourish and submitted them to me with a countenance, suggesting that he was not yet entirely sure whether he had not committed a solecism."

The professor of pathology made an impression of deep melancholy combined with bored nonchalance. Key thought that this professor looked as if he could have achieved something and as if he were mourning that such had not been the case. He gave away "a small dissertation dating from 1863, since which time he has probably not become unnecessarily involved with typesetters and printers."

The universities in Padua and Pisa did not arouse Key's interest. In Pisa he only met "a sleepy old beadle, who initiated me into the mysteries of this seat of learning."

Impressions from Some German Universities

In Germany, Key was impressed by the high salaries and standard of living of the professors, making comparisons with his own financial worries that he said "gnaw and gnaw away at the substance of one's power of thought and one's ardor . . . but—courage! Let me not give way to pathos in my letter." In Freiburg he was received by Paul Langerhans and the surgeon Vincenz Czerny, who devoted a whole day to him, after which he was invited to a large dinner with the whole faculty assembled.

The next stop was Göttingen, where Key was curious to meet Henle, whom he calls, "the foremost anatomist of our time, who is in the process of publishing the best anatomy in existence." He tells how Henle explained that it was a most extraordinary coincidence that his Swedish colleague should come on a visit at this moment, since he himself was in the process of reading a work of Key's on the kidneys. This work was of great interest to Henle; he wished to use it for the new edition of his anatomy that he was in the process of publishing. Henle stated that he had happened upon Key's work at an auction. This appears to have been an artless subterfuge, since Key was quite certain that he had sent the book to his colleague "who," he explained, "like many Germans, extracts tidbits and even steals plates for his own textbooks, which has greatly vexed me."

Back Home in Stockholm

In January 1873, Key was back in Stockholm. He was highly satisfied with the results of his journey, particularly as he had succeeded in gaining considerable publicity for *Nordiskt Medicinskt Arkiv* (*Nordic Medical Archives*). Key became the editor of this journal for a period of almost 30 years.

When asked how he was able, with a home and family, to take his leave and go gadding about the world, Key replied, "Sometimes it is as if an unavoidable fate took hold on one's life. It is as if one heard a commanding voice giving the irresistible call: You shall, you must . . . Thus this journey, for me, takes on the aspect of an imperative necessity; I feel how it is going to exert a great influence on my life and my work; I believe it is important for others as well, and for far wider interests than my own."

Key During the Last Quarter of the 19th Century

Key made his principal contribution to science—which concerned the central nervous system and its meninges—in collaboration with Gustaf Retzius. The monumental work of these two appeared in the years 1875-1876 under the title *Studien in der Anatomie des Nervensystems und des Bindegewebes*. It met with a wide international success, and was awarded the Prix Monthyon. Professor Jean-Martin Charcot congratulated Key in a hand written letter, which is preserved in the library of the Karolinska Institute: "C'est un ouvrage superbe et qui fait le plus grand honneur à la Médecine Suédoise" (Fig 18).

In 1879, Key published a paper in *Nordiskt Medicinskt Arkiv*: "Om svulstmetastaser inom centrala nervsystemets serösa banor" ("Tumour metastases in the cerebrospinal pathways of the central nervous system"). Fifty years later, Harvey Cushing wrote that his studies on tumor infiltration in the meninges were based entirely on this fundamental study.

Rector and Member of Parliament

Key was rector of the Karolinska Institute from 1886 until his retirement in 1897. He had already, in 1881, been elected to the Swedish Parliament as a liberal. In the autumn of 1890, he had found the burden of work that he had taken upon himself as rector of the Karolinska Institute was so heavy that he declined to stand for reelection to parliament. There, his speeches had been well received, and their interest focused on questions of culture, teaching, and hygiene. He strove successfully to emulate some of the House's foremost speakers. Among other achievements, he saved medical science from a much disliked coercion. At the professorial inaugurations, which took place during his period as rector, he lectured on various aspects of medical history in Sweden.

Key was a great patriot, eager to maintain the purity of the Swedish language, and in this he resembled Arthur Hazelius, creator of the Nordic Museum and the open-air museum of Skansen in Stockholm. At one time, the two men were collaborating so closely that Hazelius had his own latchkey to the professor's home so as to be able to profit by his

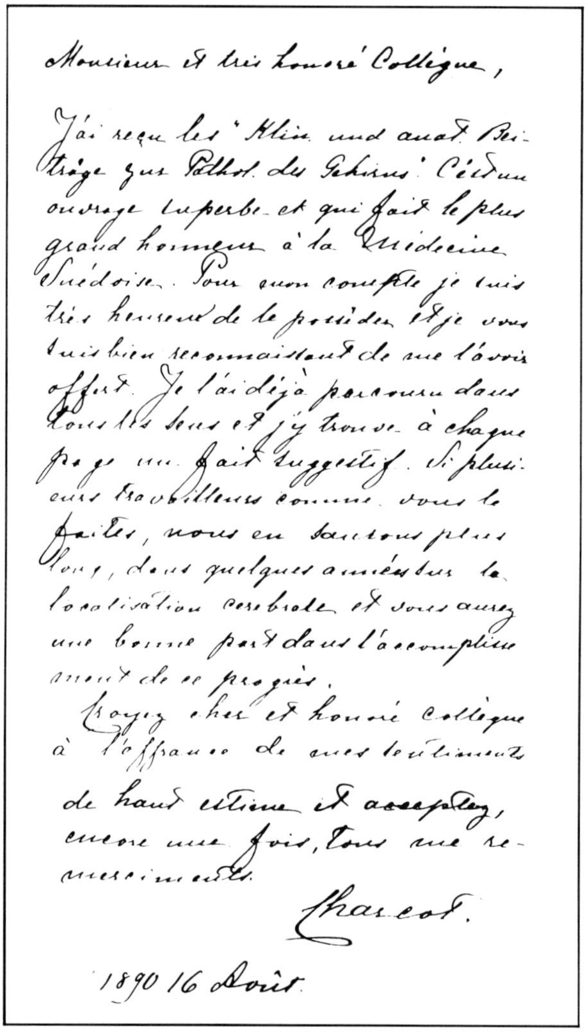

Monsieur et très honoré Collègue,

J'ai reçu les "Klin. und anat. Beiträge zur Pathol. des Gehirns". C'est un ouvrage superbe et qui fait le plus grand honneur à la Médecine Suédoise. Pour mon compte je suis très heureux de le posséder et je vous suis bien reconnaissant de me l'avoir offert. Je l'ai déjà parcouru dans tous les sens et j'y trouve à chaque page un fait suggestif. Si plusieurs travailleurs comme vous le faites, nous en saurons plus long, dans quelques années sur la localisation cérébrale et vous aurez une bonne part dans l'accomplissement de ce progrès.

Croyez cher et honoré Collègue à l'assurance de mes sentiments de haut estime et acceptez, encore une fois, tous mes remerciements.

Charcot.

1890 16 Août.

Figure 18: *Letter from Professor Charcot to Professor Key, dated August 16, 1890.*

support even at night, when Key was usually sitting up working. Hazelius' collections, which concentrated on illuminating the history of the Swedish people, had captured Key's interest at an early stage, and from 1894 Key was chairman of the Nordic Museum board. Another great project that attracted Key's attention was the University of Stockholm, which started as a seat of learning based on donations and private subscription, intended solely for work of a purely scientific nature.

Family Life in Stockholm

One of the Key daughters, in a letter to Professor Gullstrand in Uppsala, told of her childhood memories: "Mama was always sitting at her sewing-table and Papa at his desk.

The evening meal was taken at half past 8:00. That was the time when one noticed that he was in the middle of working. In contrast to the midday meal, there was not much conversation, and as soon as Papa had finished he took his second cup of tea in to his study and went on working, often until 2:00 or half past at night. For a long time, a coffee percolater was put in his study, in which he brewed up strong coffee himself during the night. I remember very clearly a time at the house on Mälartorget square, when Papa was finishing off some piece of work—I don't remember which—and he sat and wrote at his desk for two days (or three) and two nights at one stretch without a moment's sleep. There was always a boy from the printers' sitting in the hall, and he was given the manuscript in instalments as they were finished. Food was taken in to Papa on a tray, nobody was allowed to say a word, there was a lot of whispering and we crept around on tiptoe. We children thought this was terrifically exciting and we were very impressed. Mama's main feeling was probably one of anxiety. When we were grown up she often told us of how anxious she had been."

There does not appear to have been much entertaining in the Key home. Key's daughter reminisced as an adult: "A formal dinner was only given at home when some foreigner came to town. In that period, I think, this happened mainly in the summers. When Virchow made his last visit to us I was grown up. On that occasion he gave a speech, which gave me my first intimation of the degree of renown which was attached to Papa's name. This conception was then expanded and confirmed by the speech which Virchow gave in Papa's honor at the Scientific Research Congress in Munich in 1899 and by the spontaneous acclaim which was then accorded him."

Antivivisectionism in 1884

On November 25, 1884, Rickman J. Godlee resected a primary brain tumor at The Hospital for Epilepsy and Paralysis at Regents Park in London. This first operation for a primary cerebral tumor was meticulously described and well documented in the medical and popular press of the day and stimulated both professional and lay discussions of the topic that directly and indirectly led to further surgery on the cerebrum itself and the advent of modern neurosurgery. The patient died on the 28th postoperative day of secondary complications.

It is likely that only a few members of the British society took note, let alone an interest, in this landmark operation, but an active group of antivivisectionists took umbrage at this invasion of the human body and the animal experiments that made it possible. However, as a defender of the operation explained in a letter to the editor of *The Times*, "Many men and women will henceforth, there is reason to anticipate, be safe from prolonged torture and death by a kind of treatment that has been made practicable by the sacrifice, under anesthetics, of a few rabbits and monkeys." An observer of the scene later commented that this letter "ignited a controversy which raged in the columns of *The Times* for three months and evoked 64 letters and two brilliant leading articles in support of the scientific position."

In Sweden the same controversy raged, reaching the level of parliament, where the vivisection question became a matter of urgent and burning interest. A bill had been introduced that, if it were passed, would have shackled the freedom of medical research. Professor von Düben had written a statement, crushing in its arguments and extremely witty in form, that made relentless fun of the bill and had been distributed among the members of parliament. This pamphlet had aroused great bitterness among the antivivisectionists, and when the bill was read in parliament, the position was highly critical: several speakers had been playing powerfully on the feelings of the members.

Key was now in his element. His energetic manner, together with the conviction and skilfulness of his speeches, made him the master of the situation, able to dictate the decisions. This was the case in the session of 1884 in which the question of vivisection was dealt with. When Key's time came to speak, silence reigned in the chamber. The members left their seats to flock around him. He emphasized the irreplaceable value of animal experiments for research purposes in studying and combatting the epidemic diseases, pointing out the triumphs celebrated by that research. Was this now, he asked, to be cut short or be impeded in our country by inappropriate legislation, to prevent Swedish scientists from rendering their contributions to this development, of such humanitarian and cultural value? As his speech ended, a storm of applause broke out, and the bill was rejected by a large majority.

Key Meets Alfred Nobel in April 1893

In 1893, Key once more undertook a journey to foreign seats of learning. In April he arrived in San Remo. And this was the place to which Alfred Nobel had moved from Paris in 1890 after certain vexations suffered at the hands of the French authorities. When he moved to his villa in San Remo, he had taken with him his private experimental laboratory.

In the letter to his wife, dated April 19, 1893, Axel Key tells of his singular encounter with Alfred Nobel (Fig 19):

"My dearest Selma,

Yesterday, on arriving in Genoa, I was greeted by your letter of the 9th inst.—a great pleasure for me. My four days' delay has thus resulted in all the letters you have written reaching me at the place to which they were addressed. My sincere thanks.

San Remo was my last stop on the Riviera. It was a delightful day I spent there. I could have left during the afternoon, but that would have meant traversing a part of the enchanting coast road to Genoa in the dark. It was, moreover, hard to part from this place, perhaps the most charming on the whole Riviera. It was my great good fortune that I stayed. It had in any case been my intention from the outset to make a day's break there, for as you can surely imagine the journey had long been a great exertion for me: up to this point, after leaving Lyons, I had visited Nimes, Montpellier, Arles, Marseilles, Cannes, Nice, Menton, and Monte Carlo and had to each place—if I except Marseilles—devoted no more than one day, including the traveling. In sum, I stayed a further night in San Remo.

The receptionist at the hotel where I had put up had told me that Nobel, the inventor of the smokeless gunpowder dynamite etc., who had previously long been resident in Paris, had now settled in San Remo, where he had purchased a splendid villa not far from this hotel. Nobel, as you know, is a very rich man. It was he who donated 50,000 crowns to the Karolinska Institute in Stockholm. Well, at all events—I thought it would probably be pleasant to meet him—but then again, I did not want to pay him a visit that might be a bother to him and compel him to some act of politeness at an untoward moment. You know I am very anxious not to put people out.

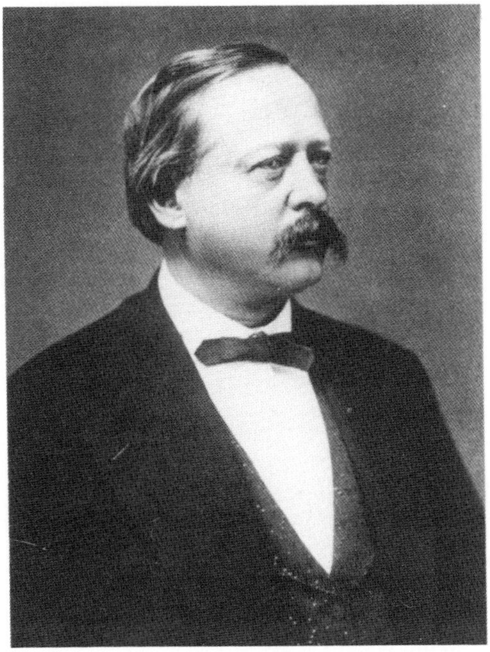

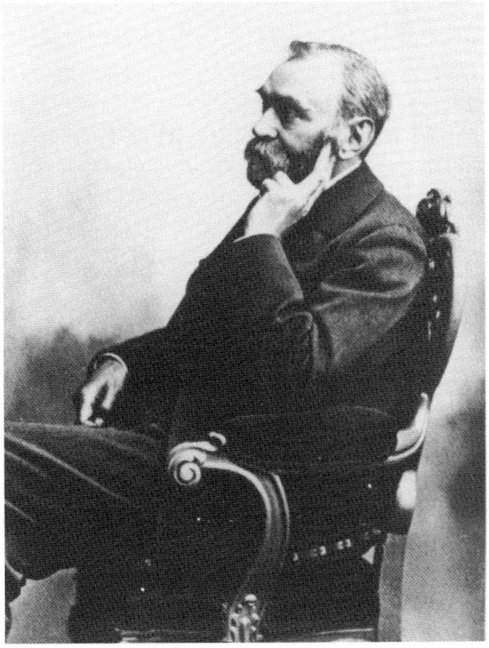

Figure 19: *Axel Key (left) and Alfred Nobel (right).*

In the afternoon I took a walk out along the road, flanked by the most splendid villas, which continues into the countryside. I had not gone far before I was struck by an exquisitely beautiful villa, quite different from any of the others and extremely impressive. I halted quite involuntarily at the gates, casting wistful looks into the splendid park that ran right down to the sea. All was so handsome and so elegant that I supposed some prince to be the happy owner of this small paradise. This conviction gained in strength when at some distance I made out the figures of two gentlemen who gave me the impression of belonging to some royal household. It was clear they did not rule the roost themselves but were rather some form of steward, or surveyors of the royal household. I was most anxious to ask them who was the owner of this enchanting villa, but they were too distant, and far too distinguished for me to hail.

A short while after, I saw the most elegant carriage drive up through the park and come to a halt before the vestibule of the villa. It was clear that a ride was soon to be taken in this fine carriage, which was of princely constitution like all else.To my delight, one of the fine gentlemen now drew near to the gate where I was standing; his aspect was so obliging and friendly that I took courage and asked him the name of the owner. Judge of my astonishment when he declared to me that it was Monsieur Nobel, and that he himself—this fine gentleman with whom I was conversing—was the concierge in office. I was seized by the wish to leave my card for Nobel, but since, as I have said, I was extremely loth to intrude upon him, I enjoined the concierge not to leave the card until after Nobel's ride, when he came home in the evening, or upon the following morning, when I was to leave at eight o'clock. He was to say that I did not wish to put Nobel to trouble but desired to pay him my respects by leaving him my card.

I then continued walking down the road; after some 30 minutes, I turned and strolled back the same way. I then found my friend, the elegant concierge, standing in the gateway. When he saw me he ran up and explained that Monsieur had enjoined him to look out for me and to show me, if I so desired, everything about the place, after which he asked for the address of my hotel. Oh! But how beautiful here this luxuriant south with its plenty, its lush vegetation—abundantly blooming camellia, orange trees bending with fruit, lemons, and luxuriant roses: everything you could imagine.

I had thought at first that Nobel had here sought a place for rest and recreation, but it was not long before my steward had led me to a splendid large laboratory which Nobel had just completed. Its equipment and all it contained showed that this was not for play but for work of the most serious kind, and the steward told me how Monsieur was ceaselessly at work. And the tasks being performed here are no mere trifles, either. This work intervenes in the fates of nations and of warfare (the smokeless gunpowder), in world industry (the production of aluminium and explosives), and then in questions of a purely scientific nature as well.

I was led out to one area, which was separated from the rest of the park by the railway, lying right beside the beach. Here, Monsieur was going to make a large winter garden. A slender iron stage led out a little way into the sea, ending in an iron platform, flanked by devices to assist bathing—but from this platform one gained the most ravishing view of the whole of San Remo. It was a view from the sea.

After a while I left this exquisite villa, and an hour later I was just about to go down to the dining room at my hotel when I was told that Nobel himself was in the hotel and insisted on meeting me. Modest, unaffected and frank, he received me in the friendliest manner. He would like to dine with me, but did not know whether he could offer me a fitting dinner in his home (he is unmarried), since in San Remo one must make one's purchases in the morning and the dinner hour had now arrived. The steward was called and asked if he could quickly arrange a suitable dinner. The answer was yes, it would take 45 minutes.

During these three-quarters of an hour, we took another extremely interesting walk in the surroundings of the villa, taking a closer view of their disposition. I had already learned something of the magnificent stables on my first visit, admiring particularly a pair of splendid black Russian horses, which were declared to be marvelously fleet. As for the iron stage below, Nobel had been granted the right to build it out into the sea by the Italian Government, a government which is highly obliged to him, having bought the patent for his smokeless gunpowder.

It grew quite dark while we were strolling round, time fled, and it seemed to me but a few minutes since I had arrived in the place when it was announced that dinner was served. Only now did we enter the villa, which until this moment had been in total darkness. As we made our way through the magnificent halls and rooms, and the verandas, the electric lighting blazed forth, and soon the entire villa and its surroundings stood thus illumined like a fairy castle. All was fine and splendid, with that solid luxury that witnesses to good, refined, and intelligent taste.

Nobel explained, 'It is not for my own sake that I arrange things thus: I could live in a hut as long as I had a good laboratory, but I need to have things done this way for the sake of all those who visit me and those with whom I must negotiate.' His whole person—simpler, even in its attire, than anyone else I saw around the place—bore out the truth of his statement.

Soon, in this fairy castle, we were sitting down to our dinner that had been arranged in 45 minutes. It was among the finest I have ever had, not by the number of dishes, though they were many, but by the supreme excellence of their preparation and by the most exquisite and select wines. After dinner, the most superb café noir and cigars with it—but what cigars!!! And excellent liqueurs and so on. (When we went for our drive I was given a whole handful of them. Smoking one now. It's good!)

When all this had been finished, accompanied by the most pleasant and interesting conversations, Nobel stated that a carriage was now at the door, if I would like to take a drive with him. I wished nothing better. I then saw that it was the black, Russian horses that were standing before a small, extremely fine phaeton; and so off we drove. The night was inky black, but a pair of splendid lamps cast a fantastic light over the immediate environs with their groves and villas—all this rushed indistinctly past in a strange and mysterious gleaming as we flew onward through the dark. We were flying, that was how I felt it—but Nobel declared that we could not give the horses free rein: the speed would not be safe in this darkness, since there was no clear view of oncoming traffic.

After a short while, I heard the sea waves breaking on one side of the road, and on the other side fantastic rocky cliffs shone out, often seeming almost to overhang us. Where are we? We are traveling along the coast road, hewn out of the rock, close by the sea, and we are heading south. In the light of the lamps we catch glimpses now of rocks, now of groves of palm and orange with their villas as we plunge onward through the coal-black night, always accompanied by the sound of the sea, far below us: between us and it there is a precipice. Suddenly, a large number of gas-lights spread out in front of us, showing that we are approaching a town. What is this? It is Hospitali, a winter resort 10 miles south of San Remo. Is it possible? I had passed the place in the train the day before, and knew that it was 10 miles from San Remo. Well! And yet we continued even further, and it seemed to me only a few moments before a sea of light once more spread out before us. This was the winter resort of Bordighera, which is yet another seven miles down the road.

Here, Nobel declared that since I was to rise the following morning at six o'clock, it was perhaps time we turned round. We stood for a long time leaning against the balustrade of the road, listening to the sound of the sea and gazing at those fantastically lighted cliffs, conducting the most lively conversation all the time. The air was marvellous, not hot enough to be oppressive, not cool enough to be chilly, but with that fresh, mild, caressing touch that is peculiar to the sea; I was going to say to the shores of the Mediterranean. Oh! How marvellous it was!

And now it was time to set off on the return journey along that captivating road, which hangs upon the cliffs as it snakes its way along the borders of the sea. Our speed increased; we seemed to fly; Nobel declared: 'Now you begin to get an idea of how these horses can travel. When it is daylight I cover 18 miles an hour with them.' I am certain this was true, for I saw that these horses were capable of our present speed with plenty to spare. We had more than 15 miles to cover. I do not know how fast we put them behind us, but I know that I could hardly believe my eyes when I saw that we were once more in the center of San Remo. We stopped at my hotel at exactly one o'clock in the morning, and here I took leave of my unexampled host.

Never shall I forget the time I spent with him. Never shall I forget that night journey, during which I could not but think of the unfortunate King Louis of Bavaria, who in the same way traveled by night in the magical illumination from his carriage, on the wild and mountainous roads of the Tyrol. This evening with Nobel has been the culmination of my journey. Nobel himself is, quite simply, an extraordinary personality and one of the most interesting acquaintances I have ever made. Imagine, then, this acquaintance being made in such surroundings and with all this background as a memory.

He was really touched, and lit up with a childlike happiness, when I showed him in a convincing manner how extraordinarily useful we found his fund. He declared once more that this fund was not the last grant with which he intended to endow the Institute. He had made further provisions in his will. It was a resplendent finish to my journey along the Riviera."

Your affectionate old
AXEL

Alfred Nobel

Nobel had devoted the whole of his adult life to work and innumerable long, exhausting journeys. He had not lived a particularly healthy life. The long exhausting journeys all over the world, irregular hours, when meals and sleep always took second place to work, had worn him down physically. He was no great devotee of festive banquets. "My demands as a rule are modest, but I do need a very good bed, because otherwise I cannot sleep, and a very good cuisine, because unfortunately I am highly dependent on it. With a stomach not finical but easily upset, I need to follow a very strict diet," he once said.

But it did once happen that Nobel was angry at not being invited to a large gala celebration. This was when the St. Gotthard Tunnel in Switzerland was inaugurated in May 1882. Dynamite, Nobel's invention, had been of decisive importance for the realization of the project, and he had not been invited to the great opening day.

Nobel was a great peace lover. He believed that his dynamite would have a deterrent effect and help to prevent war. Surely no one would wish to experience explosions of such force in battle? In a letter to the Austrian novelist and pacifist Bertha von Suttner—who was herself to be the recipient of the Nobel Prize for Peace in 1905—he wrote: "My dynamite factories can put an end to war quicker than your peace congresses. On the day when two armies are drawn up against each other in the knowledge that they can annihilate each other in less than one second, then all civilized governments will shrink from the thought of war and disband the troops." He had further developed these thoughts to Bertha von Suttner and stated to her: "I should like to invent something, an engine or a substance, to produce such horrific mass destruction that the thought of war would appear for all time to come as a manifest absurdity."

Nobel's ideas on human rationality have unfortunately not been borne out by events. The engine of destruction that he wanted to see, as an assurance for the continuation of the human race, is now a reality, but can it be claimed to have contributed to the security of human existence?

A famous doctor in Amsterdam had given his opinion that Nobel suffered from angina pectoris, while another maintained he had a severe muscular disease. He had a history of neither arterial hypertension nor transient cerebral ischemic attacks but suffered greatly from migraine headaches and serious bronchitis. The dynamite brought enormous financial success, yet Alfred Nobel was lonely and depressive. When it came to social behavior he was a typical Victorian. During dark, melancholy periods he even thought of suicide and mentioned plans to set up a mercy clinic for suicides.

When asked to write a contribution to the history of the Nobel family, Nobel after much persuasion sent the following description of himself: ". . . Alfred Nobel—a miserable half-life; should have been smothered by a compassionate doctor when he first made his crying entry into life. Greatest merits: keeps his fingernails clean and is never a burden to others. Greatest faults: has neither a family, a happy temperament, or a good stomach. Greatest and only desire: not to be buried alive. Greatest sin: refusal to worship Mammon. Important events in his life: none . . ."

During his last years, San Remo's mild and dry climate eased Nobel's discomfort. He returned to the literary interests he had had already in his youth, filling his library, which had Bjornson, Ibsen, Lie, Oehlenschläger, Hans Christian Andersen, and previously contained mostly technical books, with works of many other well-known writers. He also took up writing again. He always feared death, largely because he had a horror verging on panic of being buried alive. This was a fear that he had inherited from his father who towards the end of his life had invented a coffin with a signalling device: an occupant who had been buried alive was to be able to send out a message that he was not dead after all.

In his will, he explicitly stated that the arteries should be opened after death had been declared to ensure that he was absolutely dead. He was also afraid that he would die unattended by any personal friend. On this point his fears were tragically confirmed.

When Nobel Died

At the age of 63, Alfred Nobel on December 7, 1896, suffered a stroke—if of thromboembolic or hemorrhagic origin or even subarachnoid from a ruptured aneurysm will forever remain unanswered. He was carried to his bedroom and there, three days later, on the morning of December 10, he died attended only by an Italian doctor and some servants—just as he had feared.

It has been said that Henrik Ibsen used this brilliant, yet unhappy and tortured man as the prototype for Peer Gynt. Whether this is true or not remains unanswered, but there certainly was no Solveig or Selma waiting for him at the end.

The Testament

The temperaments of Axel Key and Alfred Nobel inclined them to self-sacrifice in the service of mankind. In February 1884 Key, who was not particularly rich, noted in his diary that, having obtained the promise of enjoying the same literary and scientific support as previously, he had undertaken at his own financial risk to continue the publication of *Nordiskt Medicinskt Arkiv*, which was in serious financial difficulties.

And Nobel, who had a distrust of lawyers, considering that they existed solely to, in his words, "prove that a straight line is in reality crooked," declared in his will that the fortune he left behind him should be used for awards—a rather imprecise formulation. One of his colleagues stated in the courtroom that Nobel had told him just before his death: "I am convinced that large inherited fortunes are an evil; they only help to make mankind dull and stupid."

Selected References

1. Brain surgery. *The Times.* November 28, 1934;15. Editorial.

2. Cushing H. Correspondence with Einar Key. Stockholm, Sweden: Karolinska Institute Library; 1929.

3. FRS. Brain Surgery. *The Times.* December 16, 1884:5. Letter to the editor.

4. Hellberg T, Jansson LM. *Alfred Nobel.* Karlshamn, Sweden: Lagerblads Publ Co; 1986.

5. Key A, Retzius G. *Studien in der Anatomie des Nervensystems und des Bindegewebes.* 1st & 2nd vols. Stockholm, Sweden: Norstedts; 1875.

6. Kirkpatrick DB. The first primary brain-tumor operation. *J Neurosurg.* 1984;61:809-813.

7. Ljunggren B, Ljunggren M. About the Nobel Prize in Medicine. *Surg Neurol.* 1987;28:331-334.

8. Ljunggren E. Axel Keys studieresa i Centraleuropa för 100 år sedan. *Yearbook of Swedish Medicine History.* Stockholm, Sweden; 1968:1-14.

9. Lundberg N. The saga of the Monro-Kellie doctrine. In: Ishii S, Brock M, eds. *Intracranial Pressure V.* Berlin, Germany: Springer Verlag; 1983:68-75.

10. Santesson CG. *Minnesskrift över Axel Key och Nordiskt Medicinskt Arkiv.* Stockholm, Sweden: Norstedts; 1932.

11. Sohlman R. *Ett testamente. Hur Alfred Nobels dröm blev Verklighet.* Stockholm, Sweden: Atlantis AB Bokförlag; 1983.

12. Strandh S: *Alfred Nobel—mannen, verket, samtiden.* Värnamo, Sweden: AB Fälts tryckeri; 1983:1-338.

13. Wallis C. Några ord till Axel Keys minne. Ett porträtt i ljustryck. *Hygiea.* 1902;64:1-10.

Chapter 4

Vladimir Bekhterev—The Professor Who Diagnosed the State of Stalin

The history of medicine is rich with innovators who have not only made important discoveries but also rendered great services to mankind. One such pioneer was Vladimir Mikhailovich Bekhterev (1857-1927), the founder of Russian neurology (Fig 20). He was a psychiatrist, a physiologist, an anatomist, a teacher, and a radical political figure—all in one person. He wrote more than 600 scientific works. The breadth of his contribution to Russian culture at the turn of the century is prodigious.

Youth

Bekhterev grew up in a village within the czarist empire, outside the city of Vyatka (now Kirov) in the administrative district of the same name. His father, a policeman, was of the impoverished rural gentry.

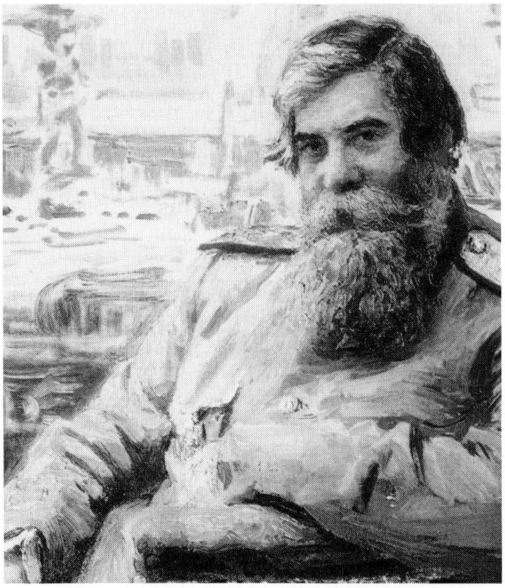

Figure 20: *Vladimir Mikhailovich Bekhterev (1857-1927) with general's rank and uniform—a portrait by Ilja Repin in 1913, the year before the Beylis trial.*

At 17 years old, Vladimir, while studying medicine in St. Petersburg (now Leningrad), was stricken with "melancholia" and admitted to the hospital for treatment. He had already been greatly influenced by the so-called nihilists of the 1860s—people who in fact held an almost religious belief in science and material progress.

He was now taken care of by Ivan Sikorsky, a young psychiatrist, who talked to him with great enthusiasm of the historic time in which they were now living—a time of new departures, when science was standing on the brink of great discoveries, particularly in the fields of brain function and the human psyche.

As Sikorsky talked with fervor on these topics, his young patient was smitten with a burning interest in psychology and brain research. By the time he was discharged from the hospital, the outline of his professional career was already mapped out.

War Experiences

When he was 20, Bekhterev interrupted his medical studies at the St. Petersburg Medico-Surgical Academy to volunteer for the Russo-Turkish War. There he was present at the historic battle of Plevna (Pleven) in September 1877, which formed a turning point of the war and initiated the retreat of the Turks after their 500 years in Bulgaria. The long battle of Plevna was fought at the price of appalling suffering and great loss of life. Bekhterev witnessed the whole action as a medic at the field hospital.

When he returned to St. Petersburg to continue his medical studies, he was a changed man. Affected by his war experiences, Bekhterev felt a stronger call than ever to use his professional work to help those in need.

Continued Studies

In 1881 Bekhterev presented a thesis on mental disturbances and their relation to body temperature. Three years later, at 27, he had 50 or more scientific articles behind him.

His teacher at St. Petersburg, Professor Ivan Merzheyevsky, now provided him with letters of introduction to some of the most highly regarded neuropathologists in Western Europe so that Bekhterev could improve himself under their tutelage. His first period of service was in Vienna under Theodor Meynert, professor of psychiatry and specialist in the structure of the cerebral cortex.

He then proceeded to Paul Emil Flechsig's famous hospital department in Leipzig. There he concentrated on studying the anatomy and cytoarchitecture of the brain stem. He made his first attempts to distinguish between different brain stem structures and a large-celled nucleus in the floor of the fourth ventricle, the upper vestibular nucleus, came to bear his name: Bekhterev's nucleus. In Leipzig, he also found time to visit Wilhelm Wundt's laboratory of experimental psychology, the first of its kind in the world.

Then, in Berlin, he worked at the Charité Hospital under its director Carl Friedrich Westphal and under the physiologist Emil Du Bois-Reymond. He concluded his tour by working under Professor Jean-Martin Charcot at the Salpêtrière Hospital.

The First Neurologist in Russia

On his return to Russia, Bekhterev, then only 28, was offered the chair of neuropathology in Kazan. He accepted on the condition that he would be given funds to follow Wundt's example by opening a laboratory of experimental physiology in association with the university.

In Kazan, Bekhterev began to work with Livery Darkshevitch (who during his time with Charcot had written an essay on brain anatomy in collaboration with the then entirely unknown Sigmund Freud). In Kazan, he devoted his entire interest to attempt to explain mental phenomena by a combination of observations on brain anatomy, physiology, and psychology.

It was he who launched the concept of neurology in Russia. He founded a publication of his own entitled *Nevrologichesky Vestnik* (*The Neurological Messenger*) and published a series of major works.

One of the things he described was a collection of nerve cells of differing sizes with a multipolar character, embedded in large numbers of nerve fibers with a net-like appearance within the brain stem—the reticular formation. He also documented nerve connections between the cerebellum and certain brain stem structures.

By the side of Ludwig Edinger, he became the first to identify the tractus spinothalamicus, the lateral fiber pathway in the anterior quadrant of the spinal cord (i.e. the afferent pain pathways in the cord that transmit pain stimuli to thalamic centers).

In addition, he demonstrated the occurrence in tabes dorsalis of an anesthetized area in the popliteal space; this became known as Bekhterev's sign.

While in Kazan, he also began to work with hypnosis, one of the subjects he had studied during his tour of Western Europe. At that time, hypnosis was regarded with great suspicion by the political power in Russia. For anyone who was to practice hypnosis in the treatment of nervous diseases, personal courage was a sine qua non—and Bekhterev had it.

Indeed, in due course he succeeded in gaining acceptance for hypnosis in his country. The hypnotic treatment that today is often used for Russian alcoholics has its roots in methods that Bekhterev introduced precisely 100 years ago. His appetite for working was enormous, and his capacity to do so amazing; he would often work into the early hours of the morning. He also married at this time, in due course becoming the father of five children.

Work on Pelvospondylitis or Ankylosing Spondylitis

In 1893, in the same year as he wrote the monograph *Provodyashchie puti golovnogo i spinnogo mozga* (*Conduction Paths in the Brain and Spinal Cord*), Bekhterev published in the *Neurologisches Centralblatt* an article entitled "Steifigkeit der Wirbelsäule und ihre Verkrümmung als besondere Erkrankungsform." The major part of this article is the translation of a report on five cases published the previous year in the Russian journal *Vrach* (*The Physician*).

In the German version, Bekhterev gives a detailed account of three cases, leaving aside two incomplete case histories from the original report in *Vrach*. The three cases were reported as exhibiting a pronounced rigidity of the cervical and upper thoracic spine. All patients showed multiple neurological disturbances with a lesion of the respiratory pathways, in all cases resulting in complete loss of intercostal breathing. The author observed atrophy and paresis in the musculature of the neck and varying degrees of muscular weakness/paresis, in one case confined to the upper extremities. There was a history of spinal traumas in two patients, one of whom had been bedridden for one month following the trauma.

In the later discussions, Bekhterev consistently maintained that these conditions differed from the disease state described by Adolf Strümpell (1884) and Pierre Marie (1898), which undoubtedly concerns cases of what today is called pelvospondylitis or ankylosing spondylitis.

At the beginning of this century, two prominent American neurologists, Sachs and Fraenkel, attacked Bekhterev for his suggestion of a disorder different from the syndrome described by Strümpell and Marie, accusing him of having invented a disease just so he could attach his name to it.

Today, pelvospondylitis or ankylosing spondylitis is well-defined. The characteristic picture is of spinal changes that typically include affection of the sacroiliac joints. There are also often extraarticular signs affecting the tendon insertions, the eyes, and sometimes the heart and lungs. The tendency to increasing stiffness is frequently pronounced, especially spinally, where the radiological picture often reveals typical bridging ossifications of the longitudinal ligaments, all resulting in a pronounced restriction of movement and usually also in a characteristic posture.

Primary pelvospondylitis is further characterized by the fact that virtually all the individuals affected have HLA (human leukocyte antigen) B 27 in their tissue type.

It was not until the present time that this typical disease picture has been more precisely defined. The diagnostic work was not seriously begun until the end of the 19th century, and the differentiation of the disease from other spinal conditions has taken a long time. Fully developed pelvospondylitis has a highly characteristic clinical picture. This has resulted in discussions on whether the disease might in fact only have made its appearance in modern times or whether it already existed in antiquity. Even in modern articles giving a broad picture of medical history, there has been a lack of clarity and a confusion between this disease and the syndrome described by Bekhterev.

The Irish physician Bernard Connor, studying in France in the 17th century, came upon a remarkable skeleton while investigating a burial ground. This skeleton exhibited total ossification and fusion of the upper part of the ilia. There was also ossification and fusion with the sacrum of a total of 15 lumbar and thoracic vertebrae and of several ribs. The general impression was of one massive, cohesive piece of bone.

Understanding the significance of this find, Connor wrote a scientific report in French, Latin, and English, this last in the form of a dissertation, which was published by the Royal Society in 1695. This paper not only gave a description, but also presented the hypothesis that the condition might be combined with pronounced restriction of movement and total dependence on diaphragmatic breathing.

Isolated reports of similar skeletal finds came during the following centuries. However, clinical descriptions were late in coming, though the question has been raised of whether Thomas Sydenham might have seen such cases in his practice.

The first to make an unequivocal connection between the pathological anatomical changes and the typical clinical picture was the English surgeon Sir Benjamin Brodie. In his textbook of 1850, he gives a clinical report of a 31-year-old man with noticeable spinal stiffness and episodes of knee joint exudation and of eye inflammation.

A few years later, the pathologist Carl von Rokitansky published good pathological anatomical descriptions, based on autopsy findings, chiefly concentrating on synostosis of the vertebral bodies and ankylosis of the intervertebral joints.

During the 1870s, a new valuable case report appeared, linking the clinical picture with the autopsy findings. The British physician Charles Fagge reported on a 34-year-old man who had gradually developed ankylosis in the rib cage, spine, and hips. When he died of bronchopneumonia, the autopsy revealed not only suppurative lung changes but also total ankylosis of the intervertebral joints.

There is no doubt that the cases published by Adolf Strümpell and Pierre Marie were cases of pelvospondylitis. In his *Lehrbuch der speziellen Pathologie und Therapie der inneren Krankheiten,* published 1884, Strümpell mentions two cases of complete spinal and sacroiliac joint ankylosis. Not until 1897 did he provide more detailed data in an article that includes a photograph of one patient.

The following year Marie published an exhaustive clinical and pathological anatomical description of the disease, which he went on to complete in later publications together with his pupil Leri. Marie emphasized the importance of ankylosis of the intervertebral joints and of the ankylosis of the root joints observed in shoulders and hips by proposing that the condition be named spondylose rhizomélique.

Bekhterev also had observed patients of the type on whom Strümpell and Marie had reported. This is made clear in an 1899 article, in which he presents two cases that he finds agree with those that Strümpell and Marie had previously described. Polemicizing against these two, he concludes the article by emphasizing that this disease—which he calls "chronic ankylosing inflammation of the major joints and the spine"—must be held separate from the spinal deformity or kyphosis in the cervical and upper thoracic spine, which he had described in 1893 and which in these cases was without exception associated with multiple neurological disturbances.

He maintained that in the patients he originally described, the peripheral joints show no changes; that neurological symptoms in the form of interrupted respiratory pathways with loss of intercostal breathing are unequivocal; that atrophy of the suprascapular and infrascapular musculature and varying degrees of weakness/paresis in the extremities are present; and that heredity, traumas, and possibly syphilis are etiological factors to be considered.

Further support for Bekhterev's view can be found in the autopsy findings of another "typical" case of Steifigkeit, which he published in direct connection with the article polemicizing with Strümpell and Marie. The illustrations in this report give the impression that the patient has advanced spondylosis and kyphosis, but there is no apparent bony bridging or block formation.

Bekhterev has stood accused as the Russian who "sowed confusion and reaped glory." However, Bekhterev's observations probably concern individuals with severe cervical and thoracic spine kyphosis secondary to, or associated with, a chronic neurological disease such as poliomyelitis, posttraumatic central cervical cord lesion, or possibly syringomyelia.

Today, pelvospondylitis is often referred to as Morbus Bekhterev, which may represent a misinterpretation of his article of 1893 entitled "Steifigkeit der Wirbelsäule und ihre Verkrümmung als besondere Erkrankungsform." This is more likely to be an early description of patients with a deformity of the spine associated with cervical cord affection and merely reveals the extraordinary acuity of Bekhterev's powers of clinical observation. As Bekhterev claimed throughout his life this syndrome has to be separated from the disease described by Strümpell and Marie.

It can hardly be doubted that competent clinicians toward the end of the 19th century were able to differentiate between typical cases of spondylosis and pelvospondylitis. Naturally, the arrival of X-ray technology made an extremely important contribution to this step forward. After 1896, several case reports on autopsy findings of pelvospondylitis were illustrated with X-ray pictures. But it was not until 1906 that a report was published concerning a patient who had had his pelvospondylitic spine examined by X-ray while alive.

Tracing out the limits between pelvospondylitis and the inflammatory rheumatic diseases, chiefly rheumatoid arthritis, was a long and wearisome process. For many years it was generally considered that pelvospondylitis was a variant of rheumatoid arthritis in which the joints of the spine were the chief focus. Earlier, in the debate concerning the difficulty of finding evidence for the occurrence of rheumatoid arthritis, the explanation had even been offered that inflammatory joint diseases during ancient times were mainly represented by pelvospondylitis and that rheumatoid arthritis only developed more recently.

In fact, the definitive conclusion of this debate did not come until the discovery in 1973 of the association of pelvospondylitis with HLA B 27, which separates it genetically from rheumatoid arthritis. Another major milestone in the differentiation of pelvospondylitis was the insight during the 1930s as to the significance of changes in the sacroiliac joints.

In his 1892 and 1893 reports, Bekhterev described neurological disturbances indicative of cervical cord lesions. These may have represented cases of syringomyelia, poliomyelitis, or posttraumatic central cord lesions associated with a pronounced cervical and thoracic spine kyphotic deformity. There is nothing to suggest that this keen clinical observer had been working with the aim of having his name associated with a certain spinal disorder. Maybe it was just an unfortunate choice to use the word Steifigkeit (rigidity) in the title of his original description of the cases with neurologic symptoms that he had observed?

Bekhterev and Russian Neurosurgery

Towards the end of 1893 Bekhterev, at 36, was inaugurated as professor at the Military Medical Academy at St. Petersburg. Here he succeeded his teacher Ivan Merzheyevsky. The significance of this advancement was that he had gained a position at the top of czarist Russian neuropathology. In association with his work at the Academy—which brought him up to the rank of general—he also took over the capital's main mental hospital and in due course a purely neurological clinic.

The first brain operation in Russia was performed in 1896. It was a case involving a cerebellar tumor that had been diagnosed by the internist Woldemar Kernig from Yurev (Dorpat). The next year, Bekhterev had a special operating theater fitted out for patients from the Military Medical Academy. Dissatisfied, however, with the results achieved in brain surgery by the prominent surgeons of the capital, he declared at the opening of his operating theater (1897): "Even if the only recourse of today's neurologists in the field of brain surgery is to untrained operators, then at least the next generation will not have to suffer such privation: for by then, specialists with neurological training behind them will have taken up the scalpel to perform what rightly forms a part of their domain."

The first "neurological surgeon" he selected was his favorite pupil, Ludvig Puusepp, age 22 and of Estonian origin. In 1899 Puusepp performed his first operation. From then on, Bekhterev consistently ignored the serried ranks of the opposing professional surgeons at the Military Medical Academy, and allowed his pupil to operate independently, though always in attendance of himself to forestall any attacks on Puusepp.

Psychoreflexology

Throughout the 1890s and during the first 10 years of the 20th century Bekhterev produced a number of writings in which he developed his reflex theory, which came to be called psychoreflexology. He analyzed mental and emotional events as expressions of neurophysiological reflex laws, coining the term associative reflexes. It is important to emphasize that there was all the while a close connection between his reflex theory and his political radicalism: if only the signals from the social environment were changed, the personality would find the power to expand and realize itself—that was the underlying concept of all that he wrote and taught.

In 1903 he commenced publication of a seven-volume encyclopedia, *Osnovy ucheniya o funktsiyakh mozga* (*Foundations of Knowledge about the Functions of the Brain*). His psychoreflexology theory was subsequently presented in the three volumes *Obyektivnaya Psikhologiya* (*Objective Psychology*) published in 1907-1910.

In more recent years, he has sometimes been called a "vulgar materialist"; it can be shown that he was a forerunner of American behaviorism. But that is far from the whole truth. He was far more complex than that: His fervent belief in man's slumbering capacities is hardly that of the behaviorist. This is the paradox of Bekhterev.

Bekhterev on Dostoyevsky

At the turn of the century some Russian psychiatrists commented on Fyodor Dostoyevsky, who had died two decades before. Writing articles on his epilepsy in professional journals, they interpreted his works entirely as the products of a sick brain. Then Bekhterev gave his own view in a lecture at St. Petersburg. He wished to give a subtler kind of picture. In this rather modest context, his statements foreshadow modern Dostoyevsky scholarship. It is important to remember that little study had been made of the novelist, who was underrated in his own country and still not well-known outside Russia.

Bekhterev spoke of Dostoyevsky's amazing psychological acuity and its prophetic qualities. He may have been the first to see the hallmark of the Dostoyevsky hero: he is a man whose every action, intention, and word is guided by one idea that has come to permeate his whole being. Raskolnikov, Ivan Karamazov, and the others are possessed by their idea. Bekhterev underlined how Dostoyevsky "clearly shows us that mentally ill and otherwise abnormal persons are not only to be found as inmates of mental hospitals but also as persons participating in everyday life together with others, the healthy ones." He emphasized that Dostoyevsky's works make it clear to us that "health and disease of the soul are so tightly interwoven in real life that it sometimes seems impossible to distinguish the one from the other."

Bekhterev's Diagnosis of Czarist Society

At the celebration of the 30th anniversary of the founding of the Military Medical Academy in December 1897, Bekhterev gave a speech that caused something of a sensation. At its outset, the address could be interpreted as being strictly professional, but it proceeded in ever sharper tones of social criticism. The speaker, taking examples chiefly from the Inquisition of the Middle Ages, showed how effective it could be to feed large masses of people with erroneous teachings, holding them down in their native ignorance and in terror, so that quite modest means—the gestures, intonation, and particular choice of words of those who had the power—were fully sufficient to guide and manipulate the masses in their apprehension of reality. The explosive power of such a speech was all the greater for its erupting within the stasis of the czarist empire.

In September 1905, the Russian psychiatrists held their second congress in Kiev. Russia had just lost the war against the Japanese, and this collapse had brought the country close to revolution. The czarist empire was shaken to its foundations. At this hour, Bekhterev chose Russian society as a subject for his diagnosis—a diagnosis of relentless clarity. The congress was hosted by Ivan Sikorsky, then one of the nation's leading psychiatrists but at the same time a man who increasingly trod the corridors of power.

Bekhterev's physical appearance alone was imposing as he stood at the rostrum: powerful and broad-shouldered, he wore a bushy and already greying beard and leveled a piercing glance at his audience. As he pronounced his condemnation of the entire czarist society, there were those among the audience who noticed a strange concordance between his figure and his words, between the power of his physical presence and his fearless political stance.

He declared, "The progress of the nation, its degree of civilization and culture, depend upon the opportunities accorded to the individual personality to develop. Whatever field of work we choose to study, we find that the active, developed personality is there enabled to scale new heights, to reach for new horizons—while the passive personality, molded by a life in slavery, is capable only of repetition and of imitation. If the personality is struggling in a slough of lawlessness, if the very spring of the nation's spiritual vitality is being sullied in this fashion—can we even speak of the strength and originality of a people?" He continued with the explicit declaration that in Russia "the personality is being strangled in its cradle by the school system, which supplies it with unusable fodder in combination with a moral repression annihilating every trace of initiative."

He stated more or less directly that the best people in Russia, those who had not allowed their native vigor to be strangled off, those who had dared to formulate "new ideas and new orders," were languishing in the prisons. The most important thing of all at this hour would be to develop the capacity for criticism and independent thought. He finished by talking of alcoholism as the curse of the Russian people and at the same time the final consequence of unfreedom.

The diagnosis was as follows: together, the Russian people form a personality, which "is being systematically repressed in family and school, which is everywhere being ensnared in routines, which is gasping for air in the vice of formalism and arbitrary despotism as in a dark and suffocating dungeon."

When at the end he quoted the lines of the poet Lermontov, "Open the prison/Bestow me with the beams of daylight," he was met by thunderous applause, as the lecture hall was entered by a squad of police and the congress had to be adjourned. Sikorsky thanked his friend with cool irony for the "service" he had rendered Russian psychiatry.

In fact, Bekhterev's fiery speech in Kiev was a manifesto. He was already nurturing plans to open his own university in St. Petersburg. This was to be financed by voluntary contributions and to contain faculties for the humanities, law, medicine, and technology. The central focus of research and teaching was to be the personality in all its manifestations. In the idea on which it was based, this university thus came to assume a revolutionary form.

By 1906, the Revolution had already been crushed and was followed by mass executions of its activists. This was the time of brutal martial law, but Bekhterev's plans lived through it. His position was so strong and his network of contacts so dense that nothing, it seemed, could stand in his way. In 1907, the plans for his Psychoneurological Institute began to assume their final shape, right in the middle of the period of czarist reaction.

A Donation

The daughter of one of the richest men in southern Russia, the owner of vast territories and a magnificent estate in the Ukraine, had committed suicide in 1906 while in a state of mental disorder; the father then decided to donate a large sum of money for the establishment of a psychiatric hospital. Not long afterward, his son also showed increasing signs of depression and growing apathy. Therefore, in the autumn of 1907, the father took the young man to his friend Bekhterev, who tried hypnosis; this seemed for a short while to exert a good effect.

What could now be more appropriate than that the donation should go to the institute whose very aim was to investigate the possibilities of developing the personality in all its facets and of removing the obstacles laid in its path by society and culture? It has been said that the funds, which soon arrived from the father of that hypnosis patient, became the final, weighty guarantee for the establishment of Bekhterev's institute. The institute was inaugurated in St. Petersburg in February 1908.

Bekhterev and Sigmund Freud

One should not be so well acquainted with the remarkable history of this donation if the son of the landed proprietor had not become the best-known psychological case of the 20th century: Sigmund Freud's classic case, the Wolf Man. Some two years after Bekhterev's hypnosis therapy, the patient, more hopelessly apathetic than ever, consulted Freud in Vienna. Four years later Freud had concluded his psychoanalytic treatment of him; after eight years the classic case description was published.

Historically speaking, it was through the Wolf Man that the paths of Freud and Bekhterev crossed for the second time. The first occasion had been their contact with Livery Darkshevitch.

Some years later (1913), they were to cross again in the collaboration with Tatiana Rosenthal, a young Russian Jewish doctor who had been won over to Freudianism. She had become a member of the Psychoanalytic Society of Vienna and had then returned to Russia and to a post at Bekhterev's institute. It was in vain that she sought to win Bekhterev to the new psychodynamic thinking from Vienna. She had imagined that Bekhterev's broad outlook, his combination of neurology and psychiatry, and his commitment to social psychology (a commitment entirely absent in Freud) would be susceptible to a cross-pollination with Freud's ideas. But she was mistaken. Bekhterev was, in the end, too mechanistic in his view of man to be able to accept depth psychology.

The Psychoneurological Institute

Tatiana Rosenthal was thrice typical of the staff recruitment at the Psychoneurological Institute. She was a woman, she was Jewish, and she was a political radical. Here, teachers and students were accepted without regard for sex, for religious beliefs (as a result of the increasing limitation on numbers admitted to universities, Jews were being largely excluded), or for political reliability (it was quite common for students to be driven away from university studies on political grounds). This was rare in Russian higher education at that time.

In fact, Bekhterev's institute was the first free university in the history in Russia. The teaching staff included several political figures who had previously been more or less banned. Perhaps the best known of these was Maxim Kovalevsky, who had returned from almost 20 years of exile and whom Bekhterev had made the country's first professor of sociology.

The World's First Professorship in Neurosurgery

In the same year that Bekhterev founded his institute, he had Ludvig Puusepp (Fig 21) appointed associate professor at the department of the Military Academy. Puusepp immediately requested permission of the academy to teach neurosurgery, but it was not forthcoming since the academy surgeons considered that he was trespassing on their domains. At this point Bekhterev responded by establishing at his institute a special Chair for Surgical Neuropathology; in 1910 Puusepp was appointed professor within this new speciality.

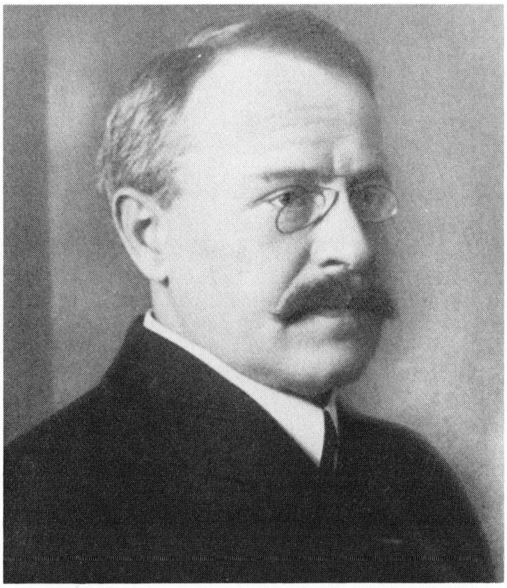

Figure 21: *The first professor of neurological surgery—Ludvig Puusepp of Estonian origin.*

It was in the same year that Harvey Cushing was offered the Chair as Professor of Neurosurgery at Washington University in St. Louis. Cushing, however, turned this down before he moved to Boston in 1912 and the chair in St. Louis was filled by Ernest Sachs, who accepted his professorship in the fall of 1910.

Puusepp and Sachs thus became the world's first professors of neurosurgery. In the classic work on the history of neurosurgery by Earl Walker it is noted: "Bekhterev realized as early as this—when Harvey Cushing was being informed by his contemporaries that he would have to go hungry if he dared to persist in his wish to establish a speciality in brain surgery that there was a need for neurologically trained operators who could perform both brain and spinal cord surgery." This was at a time when Harvey Cushing's operative mortality was some 30 percent (in the period 1901-1912) for the most common brain tumor type, the glioma.

Puusepp also emphasized in his memoirs the fact that Bekhterev alone, before anyone else, realized the necessity of training specialist neurosurgeons, in the face of deep skepticism on the part of the medical establishment. Soon after the seizure of power by the Bolsheviks, Puusepp moved to the University of Tartu (Dorpat). His departure from Petrograd left a vacuum in Soviet neurosurgery that remained unfilled for more than a decade.

Bekhterev and Ivan Pavlov

When Puusepp was appointed professor of neurosurgery, he was 35. He had started his career under Ivan Pavlov (Fig 22), who was also working in St. Petersburg. After a while, Puusepp had transferred to Bekhterev's institute, but he always retained a deep respect for his first teacher. Although Pavlov was eight years Bekhterev's senior, the careers of the two men had otherwise run almost parallel. They came from modest circumstances and

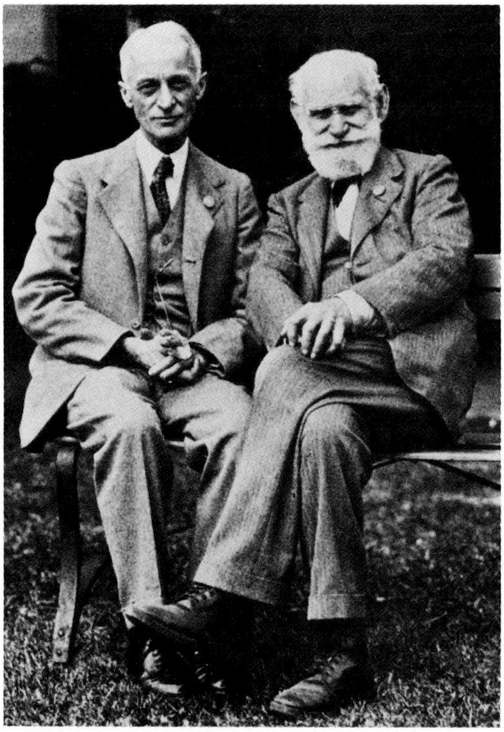

***Figure 22:** Harvey Cushing and Ivan Pavlov.*

they had made their study trips to the West at almost the same time. Each had opened his own research laboratory in the capital of czarist Russia, focussing on neurophysiology. Though researching within walking distance of each other, each developed his own reflexology. They might almost appear to be each other's doubles, though they were fundamentally different as research personalities. Pavlov was the deeper and more concentrated of the two, Bekhterev the broader and more multifaceted.

It is one of the ironies of history that they became each other's enemies, since—as Puusepp emphasized in his memoirs—they could have excellently complemented each other, to the benefit of Russia and of all mankind.

Their enmity took shape soon after the turn of the century, when Bekhterev began publication of his vast brain encyclopedia; this was reviewed by Pavlov, who began by calling it "unique in world literature" and then went on to subject it to detailed criticism of a heavy-handed and entirely insensitive nature. A real struggle for power developed between the two. Thus Bekhterev spoke of associative reflexes instead of Pavlov's conditioned reflexes. He performed his experiments on humans where Pavlov worked with animals. His interest centered on the function of the brain and on human behavior, while Pavlov was studying the purely physiological reactions. It need hardly be pointed out that the future belonged to Pavlov, his results being so much more concrete, so much easier to measure exactly. However, this still allows us to establish the fact that Bekhterev and his psychoreflexology have made important contributions to present neurology.

The enmity between Bekhterev and Pavlov was so pronounced that they would insult each other in the street. If they ran into each other at the same congress they would soon be embroiled in dispute. Forming cliques and slinging snide shots at each other, they were engaged in a constant struggle to expose one another's faults and weaknesses. No sooner had some pupil of Bekhterev made a public statement than it was parried by Pavlov's retort—which followed virtually as a conditioned reflex.

Puusepp rightly points out in his memoirs that on these occasions Pavlov's efforts were far from always crowned with success; there were times when the component of private vengefulness was all too obvious. Whenever a disciple of Pavlov made a pronouncement, Bekhterev was ready with an attempt to repudiate his argument, and often with poor results, since his own contribution to the debate was so clearly aggressive and aimed at the person.

Patriot and Pan-Slavist

In his view of society, Bekhterev was above all a patriot. He kept his distance from politicizing and did not belong to any revolutionary party. It was the fate of Russia that worried him, the backwardness of the Russian nation, and the miseries of the Russian people. In accordance with his patriotism, he found himself becoming committed to the cause of Pan-Slavism, the dream of the unification of Slavic cultures that was so vivid at the beginning of this century. In fact he had really been a Pan-Slavist from early youth and his experiences during the Bulgarians' struggle for freedom from the Turks had strengthened his feeling of Slavic brotherhood.

In 1909, he took part in arranging an international Pan-Slavic congress in St. Petersburg. The following year he traveled to a similar congress in Sophia (the capital of Bulgaria), taking the opportunity to revive his memories of the battle of Plevna. Two years later, Tomás Masaryk hosted the Pan-Slavic congress in Prague with Bekhterev among the guests.

Masaryk had also succeeded in firing the enthusiasm of the aging Leo Tolstoy for the Pan-Slavic idea, but shortly afterward, in the autumn of 1910, the latter died while fleeing his aristocratic life on his estate of Yasnaya Polyana. The course of his death struggle at the railway station of Astapovo was followed by the whole nation, and many felt that it was as if Russia were floundering together with the aged prophet and truth-teller.

Bekhterev, who held Tolstoy in great admiration, showed poor judgment at that moment by sending a telegram for Tolstoy's brain even before he was dead. Tolstoy's relatives as well as his admirers felt deeply hurt by Bekhterev's action. Maybe the shocking outspokenness of it should be seen just as one expression of Bekhterev's utter frankness in all he undertook.

Bekhterev's New Challenge

At the beginning of September 1911, partly on the initiative of Ivan Sikorsky, the first conference of the newly founded Russian Society of Psychiatrists and Neuropathologists was held in Moscow. At that time, Russia was in a state of deep political depression and social change seemed farther off than ever.

A few months previously, more than 100 professors and lecturers had resigned from the University of Moscow in protest against the repressive policy of the Ministry of Education; among these teachers were several colleagues and friends of Bekhterev's. The listlessness of young people had led to veritable epidemics of suicide; decadent "suicide clubs" had sprung up in several cities.

In his address at the conference, Bekhterev took it upon himself to try to expose the sociopsychological causes of this frightening spread of suicide. Every word he uttered was noted down by an agent of the police in the audience, and the transcript has been preserved in the unusually thick dossier on Bekhterev, which was found in the Okhrana archives after the Revolution. "One of the main causes of the suicides," he declared, "is to be found in the conditions currently obtaining in the Russian schools. These schools are now turning out tortured neurasthenics . . . the schools are sunk in darkness—they must be changed. It is the murky elements of the night who have produced this darkness, trampling upon the best of our social and human ideals. It is now up to us to teach young people to stand firm against these misfortunes and not to yield to pessimism."

There was a move to break off the conference at that point, but Bekhterev escaped with a warning from the police officer, which is especially remarkable for the fact that he had already begun the conference with an unheard-of challenge. Some days before, the Russian Prime Minister Piotr Stolypin had been assassinated at the Opera in Kiev. One minute's silence had been ordained in memory of the dead man at the opening of the conference, and all the delegates were to stand. All present rose to their feet—except for the chairman, Bekhterev, who remained demonstratively seated. He had not forgotten Stolypin's mass executions in the wake of the failed Revolution of 1905.

Bekhterev's police dossier increased in thickness and his enemies in number. The dossier reveals that Stolypin had made arrangements for "serious attention" to be directed at all that went on within the walls of the Psychoneurological Institute. And in the margin of one police report the czar himself had noted, "Of what use is this Institute to Russia? Kindly produce a well-founded reply." However, Bekhterev was not an easy prey: He was the leading figure of the nation's psychiatry, he was an army general and—perhaps most important—he appears already at this stage to have been secretly treating the czaritza for hysteria. Powerful opponents he did have, but he also had powerful friends.

Two Murders in Kiev

In Kiev in 1911, there occurred two murders that were to have consequences for the 20th century history of Russia. In September, the most forceful politician of the czarist empire, Stolypin, was shot. Previously to that, a 13-year-old, Andrey Yushchinsky, was the victim of an atrocious murder. His dead body, mutilated by 50 stab wounds, was found in a cave.

Rumors soon began to circulate that the boy had fallen victim to Jews committing a ritual murder before drinking his blood. A person in a high position is said to have seen to it that these unfounded rumors gained wide circulation. They duly resulted in violent anti-Semitic campaigns, in the same pattern as when the pogroms 10 years earlier had swept the Ukraine. This was a convenient way for the authorities to distract attention from the social discontent in the country; once more the lot could fall upon the Jews as scapegoats.

In actual fact, it seems likely that Yushchinsky had been removed from the scene because, after helping a band of robbers wanted by the authorities, he had threatened to reveal all he knew to the police. Shortly after, a peaceable Jewish accountant at a brickyard in Kiev, Mendel Beylis, was arrested and brought to trial as a ritual murderer.

The End of a Long Friendship

Ivan Sikorsky, the pride of Kievan psychiatry, was then brought on stage, where he lent himself to an expert pronouncement, in which instead of freeing Beylis from guilt, he made it clear that the many knife thrusts might have been connected with a ritual murder involving the drinking of the victim's blood.

One may wonder how Sikorsky, being one of the most respected healers of mental illness in Russia, could allow himself to be used and lend his signature to such a document. He may have been grieved that he had not got further professionally and that he had not realized more of the great dreams he once had. He had increasingly become an errand boy of power. For instance, he had seen to it that young men who refused to bear arms on the basis of their membership of various religious sects were certified as mentally ill. This brought him on a collision course with Bekhterev, who by various temporizing expedients was trying to save the students of the Psychoneurological Institute from military service.

To Bekhterev, Sikorsky's expert pronouncement came like a bolt from the blue. He had hoped to maintain his respect for, and his friendship with, the man who once had guided him onto the psychoneurological track, but now it was no longer possible. And in those same months, anti-Semitic feelings were being stirred up all over Russia with the approaching trial of Mendel Beylis. These feelings culminated in excesses of propaganda, which are reminiscent of Nazi Germany (right-wing extremist magazines were speaking of Jews as reptiles that must be exterminated). Bekhterev was bringing his guns to bear for the counterattack.

The Russian Dreyfus Affair

In 1912, when Mendel Beylis had already spent a year in prison, Bekhterev brought together the psychiatric authorities of the Western world to form a "counterexpertise" to Sikorsky's pronouncement. Their white book (official government report) came out in Germany in early 1913 under the title *Der Fall Justschinski*. Its contributors were Eugen Bleuler, Karl Bonhöffer, Julius Wagner-Jauregg, Heinrich Obersteiner, Auguste Forel, Ernst Meyer, and other well-known specialists in psychiatry and neurology. Their judgment was unanimous and harsh. Wagner-Jauregg, head of the famous University Hospital of Vienna, found it "incredible" that a psychiatrist—and a respected one at that—should lend his name to something of this nature. Meyer, a professor in Königsberg, noted that he had read the implausibilities of Sikorsky's pronouncement "with deep concern."

In the early days of August 1913, the 17th International Medical Congress was held in London. The 7,000 delegates included many of the greatest contemporary figures in medicine, surgery, and psychiatry. They included Harvey Cushing, Pierre Janet, and Carl Gustav Jung—and they included Bekhterev, who now mobilized the entire congress to a powerful protest against the expert pronouncement of Sikorsky.

In the autumn of the same year, Bekhterev was summoned as an expert witness at the trial. His friends warned him not to travel to Kiev, but he never hesitated. His great single combat not only with Sikorsky but with czarism in general was approaching its climax, just as the Romanov dynasty was celebrating the tercentenary of its reign. With the *Der Fall Justschinski* behind him, Bekhterev now succeeded in tearing Sikorsky's pronouncement to shreds and thus annihilating one of the major foundations of the case against Beylis. Incisively, he laid bare its encapsulated political prejudice with all its embarrassing lack of scientific professionalism.

The aging Sikorsky seemed to have been almost incapable of entering a defense. At first he was unwilling even to appear in court; once there, he lost the thread of his argument, stuttered, repeated himself, and strayed from his subject. He declared, for instance, that Russia was under threat of destruction since "a canine pack of bankers, doctors, and sexual psychopaths" (i.e. all Jews) were tenaciously working to bring an end to the nation. The trial climaxed in what no one had expected: the Jewish accountant was acquitted for lack of evidence. Czarist power had ordered a conviction—but the skillful defense lawyers, together with Bekhterev, had broken all resistance.

A few years later Sikorsky died, at almost the same time as Imperial Russia fell. This Russian Dreyfus affair may in fact be seen as in some way forming the starting point of the revolutionary process. It revealed the spread of the internal decay in that social system. And this is indeed the way it is portrayed, half a century later, by the American author Bernard Malamud (himself born of Jewish parents in Kiev a few months after the conclusion of the trial) in his novel *The Fixer.*

It is symptomatic that the French newspaper *La Libre Parole*, which played such a fateful role in the Dreyfus affair, heaped words of contumely on Bekhterev after the Kiev trial. He was pictured as a subversive freemason, working in collusion with the Jews to overthrow the social order.

Bekhterev's Punishment

Bekhterev paid for his courage. He was removed from office as director both of the Psychoneurological Institute and of the Military Medical Academy (where his workload had been so heavy that he now had to be replaced by two full-time professors). His enemies used all the means at their disposal to annihilate the Institute, which in their eyes was nothing but a focus of antisocial infection. They finally succeeded in March 1917, three days before the Revolution came.

When the Bolsheviks seized power in the autumn of 1917, Bekhterev, having hitherto professed no political allegiance, took their side. He was first of all a patriot and under no circumstances did he wish to go into exile. In 1918, he opened a brain institute in Petrograd, and soon he was working as actively as ever.

Bekhterev and Luriya

In a manner of speaking, the paths of Freud and Bekhterev crossed once more in the 1920s. In 1922, a 19-year-old student, Aleksandr Luriya, started a psychoanalytical seminar in Kazan. He sent a report of this activity to Freud. This communicative young man soon also turned his interests to the psychology that was in fashion in the Soviet state and to psychoreflexology.

He went to Petrograd to suggest to Bekhterev that they should work together. Bekhterev was impressed by Luriya's enterprising spirit. After a few months together, they published a journal with the ambitious title: *Voprosy psikhofiziologii, gigieny truda i refleksologii* (*Questions of Psychophysiology, Work Hygiene and Reflexology*). It was printed on rejected wrapping paper from a soap factory in that period of acute paper shortage, and only two issues, now considered bibliographical rarities, were published.

Luriya was aiming to work out "a reflexological method for researching into suggestibility"; Bekhterev contributed articles that formed part of his attempt to bind the theory of reflexology closer to Marxism. Luriya, however, developed in a direction leading away from his teacher. He became the best known Russian psychologist of this century and the founder of the new scientific discipline of neuropsychology, which was developed in close collaboration with Soviet neurosurgeons. In one essential respect he always remained Bekhterev's pupil—in his attempts to relate mental processes to brain physiology.

When Bekhterev's Fate Was Sealed

Ten years after the Revolution, in December 1927, the 70-year-old Bekhterev was called to the Kremlin by Joseph Stalin. Three years after the death of Lenin, Stalin was engaged in the final stages of the struggle for power, his main adversaries being Trotsky and his adherents. Stalin felt depressed. There was nothing strange in his turning to Bekhterev, for the latter was the undisputed psychoneurological authority in the Soviet state and he had also rendered the Revolution "exceptional services." In 1923, the ailing Lenin had twice sent for him.

It is unclear, as perhaps it will always remain, what then ensued. Persistent rumors in the Soviet Union have it that Bekhterev diagnosed Stalin as suffering from "grave paranoia." The same day he had visited the Kremlin he suddenly died. According to the rumors, Stalin had him murdered, this being the patient's revenge for the diagnosis. There is much to suggest that this may really be what happened.

In the early 1980s, the rumors about Bekhterev's death appeared to find corroboration in the memoirs of Lidiya Shatunovskaya, released in the West under the title *Zhizn v Kremle* (*A Life in the Kremlin*). At the time in question, Shatunovskaya had been living in the Kremlin with her husband, a high party official who later, like his wife, was sent to a camp. The author claims that the course of events was that described in the rumors.

Bekhterev's frank pronouncements and the revenge of the despot would entirely agree with what is known today of these two personalities. Bekhterev feared no one: throughout his life he had stared power straight in the face and spoken his mind without prevarication. He had been in the best of health in the days before he suddenly died. Curiously, postmortem was never held; his body was cremated in accordance, it was said, with his wish expressed shortly before his death.

In his memoirs noted down by Solomon Volkov, Dmitry Shostakovich also brings up these rumors. He refers to his family doctor, the surgeon Grekov, declaring his conviction that Stalin was "mad." It appears that Grekov, who was a friend of Bekhterev's, related one day in Shostakovich's home that Bekhterev was one day "called to the Kremlin, where he made a careful examination of Stalin's mental condition. He died just afterwards, and Grekov was certain that Bekhterev had been poisoned."

New facts, presented in a pseudonymous work by the Soviet historian N. Petrenko in 1986, reveal that shortly after his death Bekhterev was replaced as head of the Brain Institute by one of his pupils, Viktor Osipov. The latter appears to have been Stalin's henchman, attempting in various ingenious ways during the sickness of Lenin to cast doubts upon Lenin's mental condition, against the background of Lenin's increasing malaise at the suggestion of Stalin being given a leading post after his death.

Once Stalin had taken power into his own hands, Bekhterev's scientific work was subjected to growing criticism, at the same time as Ivan Pavlov was being raised to the status of a national monument. Bekhterev's work was not republished for 40 years. Most of the indications suggest that Bekhterev had met one who was more than a match for him when he ran across the bloodiest tyrant of Russian history—that he thus became one of the latter's first victims.

Today, psychohistorical dissertations are being written on Stalin, showing how his pathological personality appears in the 1930s to have plunged the entire Soviet Union into a state of collective psychosis. Millions were murdered as enemies of the people because the despot, as it seems, was suffering from a persecution mania. Maybe the simple fact is that Bekhterev was the first to make the correct diagnosis of him.

Under *glasnost*, writers and historians in the Soviet Union have recently dared with increasing frequency and frankness to question the dictator's state of mental health. The philosopher Dmitry Volkogonov, who is preparing the first official biography of Stalin, reflected in an article in *Literaturnaya Gazeta* in 1987, "Was there not, beside Stalin's cruelty, a mental illness never clarified? In the absence of this, it is hard to explain why, once he had eliminated his rivals, he had to go on 'cutting down' the best men of the Party and the State in the very hour of desperate adversity" (i.e. the defensive war against the Germans).

Volkogonov would be able to cite a statement of Marshal Zhukov, made to the author Jelena Rzhevskaya. According to a memorial essay in the journal *Znamya* (*The Flag*) Zhukov, one of the few who was at all close to Stalin, told Rzhevskaya that Stalin had said in 1946, "I am the unhappiest of men. I even live in fear of my own shadow."

An article in the *Literaturnaya Gazeta* (September 1988) entitled "The Last Diagnosis—A Most Probable Version, Which Deserves Further Research" explained that Bekhterev's son Pyotr was convinced that his father had been poisoned. Later Pyotr suffered a similar fate—he was shot by order of Stalin. Other Bekhterev descendants like his granddaughter Natalya Bekhtereva, professor of neurophysiology in Leningrad, hold the same opinion regarding Vladimir Bekhterev's ultimate fate.

In the same article, Andrej Lichko, professor of psychiatry and vice-head of the Psychoneurological Institute, described how Stalin's paranoia was of a cyclic type occurring at intervals like the waves of persecutions that went over Russia first in 1929 to 1930, then in 1936 to 1937, and finally toward the end of Stalin's life when new processes were planned against Jewish doctors.

In the Soviet weekly *Ogonyok* (1988), Mikhail Fromm, a well-known film director, has reported his memories from the Khrushchev era. In a speech to about 650 Soviet intellectuals, Khrushchev, according to Fromm, had said about Stalin: "Do you think that we had an easy life back in those days. To be honest (Khrushchev lowered his voice and it seemed as if he had just forgot that he had a large auditorium) between us, he was insane during his last years, INSANE with total control over the whole society, can you imagine. . . ."

In today's perspective, Bekhterev appears as one of the broadest and most colorful personalities that Russia has ever produced. Nothing can be said for certain, but there is much evidence that Stalin ordered the murder of this fearless speaker of unpleasant truths once the diagnosis of "grave paranoia" had been pronounced. It appears most likely that Bekhterev, for the first time in his life, had here encountered one who was more than a match for him.

Postscript

Ernst Kretschmer in a letter to Oswald Bumke (1933) wrote, "It's a funny thing about psychopaths. In normal times we render expert opinions on them. In times of political unrest they rule us."

Selected References

1. Bekhterev VM. *Die Leitungsbahnen im Gehirn und Rückenmark; Ein Handbuch für das Studium des Nervensystems* [in Russian]. Leipzig, East Germany; 1894.

2. Bekhterev VM. *Obyektivnaya psikhologiya.* 1st-3rd vols. St Petersburg, USSR; 1907-1910.

3. Bekhterev VM. *Osnovy ucheniya o funktsiyakh mozga.* 1st-7th vols. St Petersburg, USSR; 1903-1907.

4. Bechterew W. Neue Beobachtungen mit pathologisch-anatomischen Untersuchungen über Steifigkeit der Wirbelsäule. *Deutsche Zeitschrift für Nervenheilkunde.* 1899;15:45-57.

5. Bechterew W. Steifigkeit der Wirbelsäule und ihre Verkrümmung als besondere Erkrankungsform. *Neurologisches Centralblatt.* 1893;12:426-434.

6. Bechterew W. Über ankylosierende Entzündung der Wirbelsäule und der grossen Extremitätengelenke. *Deutsche Zeitschrift für Nervenheilkunde.* 1899;15:37-44.

7. Bechterew W. Über die innere Abteilung des Strickkörpers und den achten Hirnnerven. *Neurologisches Centralblatt.* 1885;3:145-147.

8. Brazier MAB. The great Russian schools explore the field of neurophysiology. In: Brazier MAB, ed. *A History of Neurophysiology in the 19th Century.* New York, NY: Raven Press; 1987:212-248.

9. Bywaters EGL. Historical introduction. In: Moll JMH, ed. *Ankylosing Spondylitis.* London, England; 1980:1-15.

10. *Der Fall Justschinski: Offizielle Dokumente und private Gutachten.* Berlin, Germany; 1913.

11. Guberman IM. *Bekhterev: Stranitsy Zhizni.* Moscow, USSR; 1977.

12. Käbin I. Die Medizinische Forschung und Lehre an der Universität Dorpat/Tartu 1802-1940. Ergebnisse und Bedeutung für die Entwicklung der Medizin [in Swedish]. *Sydsvenska Medicinhistoriska Sällskapet.* 1986;6(suppl).

13. Lobner H, Levitin V. A short account of Freudism. Notes on the history of psychoanalysis in the USSR. *Sigmund Freud House Bulletin.* 1978;1:5-30.

14. Moroz O. Poslednij diagnoz pravdopodobnaya versiya, trebuyushchaya, odneko, dalneyshey proverki. *Literaturnaya Gazeta.* 1988;Sept 28:12.

15. Ott V. Bechterew's syndrome—A historical review. In: Proceedings from a symposium on Bechterew's syndrome and allied disorders. *Scand J Rheumatol.* 1980;32(suppl):7-13.

16. Petrenko N. Lenin v Gorkach—bolezn i smert (Istochnikovedcheskie zametki). In: Minuvsheye. *Istorichesky almanakh.* Paris, France; 1986:143-287.

17. Raudam E, Kaasik AE. Ludvig Puusepp 1875-1942. In: *Neurosurgical Giants: Feet of Clay and Iron.* New York, NY: Elsevier; 1985:283-287.

18. Rzhevskaya E. V tot den, pozdnej osenyu. *Znamya.* 1986;12.

19. Sachs B, Fraenkel J. Progressive ankylotic rigidity of the spine (Spondylose Rhizomélique). *J Nerv Ment Dis.* 1900;27:1-15.

20. Shatunovskaya L. *Zhizn v Kremle.* New York, NY; 1982.

21. Thomson AF. Ludvig Puusepp 1875-1942. In: Walker E, ed. *A History of Neurological Surgery.* Baltimore, Md: Williams & Wilkins; 1951:270-271.

22. Volkogonov D. Fenomen Stalina. *Literaturnaya Gazeta.* 1987;Dec 9.

23. Volkov S. Testimony. In: Volkov S. *The Memoirs of Dmitri Shostakovich.* New York, NY: Harper & Row; 1979.

24. The Wolf-Man: Recollections of my childhood. In: Gardiner M, ed. *The Wolf-Man and Sigmund Freud.* London, England; 1973:3-132.

25. Yakovlev PI. Vladimir Mikhailovich Bekhterev (1857-1927). In: Haymaker W, ed. *Founders of Neurology.* Springfield, Ill: Charles C Thomas Publisher; 1953:244-247.

Chapter 5

The Case of General Leonard Wood

Reprinted by permission of *Journal of Neurosurgery*.

Leonard Wood, major general and chief of staff of the United States Army, was a military surgeon turned career officer (Fig 23). There were many romantic tales from the American Indian wars that surrounded his name.

In the summer of 1897, he became acquainted with Theodore Roosevelt. After the meeting the future president, Roosevelt, enthusiastically wrote to his wife, "In the evening I dined with the Lowndes who were just dear. There was a very interesting Dr. Wood of the army there; he had been all through those last Apache campaigns, which were harassing beyond belief."

A Regrettable Mishap

After a spell as military governor of Cuba, Wood had entered the forefront of the contemporary political scene. In the autumn of 1898, he had been unlucky enough to strike his head against a low-hung chandelier with such force that he was confined to his bed for a full week after the accident.

Later, Wood became aware of an exostosis, slowly increasing in size, at the site of the trauma to the cranium, which was on the crown of the head just to the right of the midline. By 1902, there was a sensation of numbness on the outside of the left foot and, in November 1904, Wood experienced a sudden spasmodic attack beginning in the left foot, running up the leg, and reaching the muscles of respiration. He did not lose consciousness. After that he had many slight similar attacks.

In 1905, Wood was operated on for a tumor projecting from the calvaria just to the right of the median line. The tumor was found to be of the psammomatous variety, a soft tumor with a shell of bone, and pressing upon the dura. It was not discovered at this operation that any part of the tumor projected within the dura.

Harvey Cushing Takes on the Case

In January 1909, Wood, then 48 years old, was referred to Dr. Harvey Cushing at The Johns Hopkins Hospital in Baltimore by Dr. Arthur Tracy Cabot because of increasing left-sided Jacksonian attacks with slight postictal motor deficits. Since 1895, Cushing had been particularly interested in the meningiomas and had become increasingly convinced that they were a particular type of brain tumor, with a more favorable prognosis than most of the others.

Even by 1909, however, only an occasional successful operation on an intracranial meningioma had been reported in the literature. It was not until 1922 that Cushing himself, in an article in the periodical, *Brain*, coined the term *meningioma* for this type of benign brain tumor. Previous to this, meningiomas had been known by a bewildering variety of terms—including dural endothelioma, fungoid neoplasia of the dura mater, meningeal fibroblastoma, and arachnoid fibroblastoma—and it had not been clearly understood how to differentiate them from the sarcomas.

General Wood's Operation

When Cushing had examined Wood at The Johns Hopkins in January 1909, it was apparent to him that the tumor extended intracranially as well, close to the midline. At first Cushing adopted a conservative attitude, recommending a policy of "wait and see" until such time as surgery might be indicated. There was as yet scanty experience of operations on this type of lesion; in fact, no experience at all of benign midline growths, later to be classified as parasagittal meningiomas. Moreover, the diagnosis of a suspected brain tumor at this time still relied entirely on clinical findings. The important diagnostic aids of cerebral angiography and ventriculography had not yet been discovered.

However, during the autumn of 1909, Wood's condition deteriorated, and in February 1910, Cushing therefore made the decision to attempt surgery. The operation was carried out in two stages, at an interval of four days: at the second stage, Cushing had only to raise the bone flap, which had been sawed out on the first occasion. The dura was opened to expose the surface of the brain in the vicinity of the tumor. There were clear signs of raised intracranial pressure. The tumor was plainly visible just at the border of the sagittal sinus, and Cushing at first took it to be a glioma. However, as he worked his way

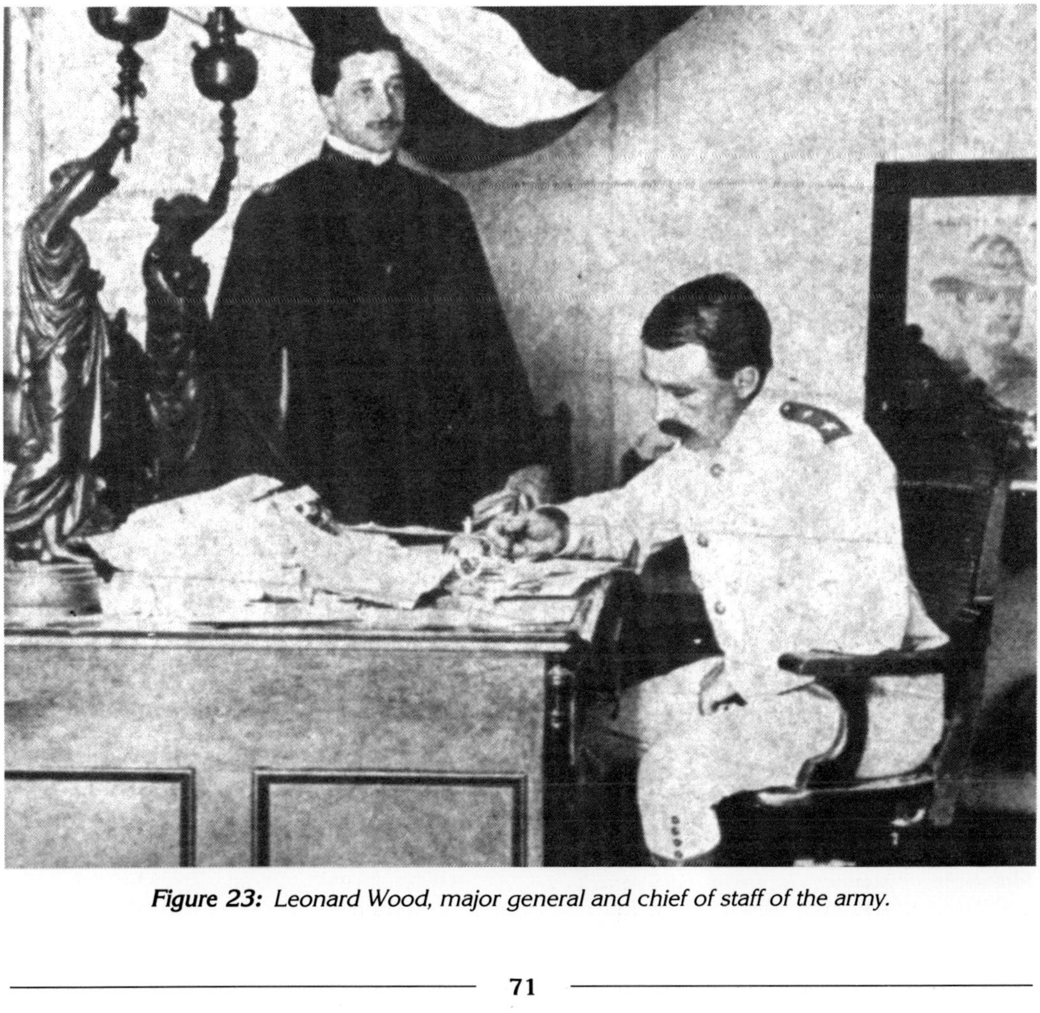

Figure 23: *Leonard Wood, major general and chief of staff of the army.*

down in the hemisphere in the plane of demarcation between the tumor and the surrounding parenchyma, it became clear that the limits of the growth were quite clear even to the naked eye. Cushing meticulously dissected in the plane of demarcation, and was able to achieve at last what appeared to be a complete extirpation of the whole tumor, sparing the bridging veins both in front of and behind the area affected by the tumor.

The patient stood up well to surgery, walking around on the 11th day after the operation. He was discharged from The Johns Hopkins Hospital after scarcely a month had passed, at which point he felt his recovery to be virtually complete, and resumed his previous occupations with undiminished vigor.

This was the first time that Cushing had successfully operated on an intracranial meningioma. With the vascularity of such tumors (compare Vilhelm Magnus' opinion on this subject, see Chapter 2) in mind, one can imagine that the technical obstacles encountered probably were considerable, working as Cushing did with the primitive anesthesia techniques and operating equipment of his time.

The operation on Wood represented the turning point for Cushing in his career as a neurosurgeon. The successful removal of the parasagittal meningioma from the U.S. Army chief of staff doubtless helped to secure for Cushing the Moseley Chair of Surgery at Harvard University in 1912 and with it the post of surgeon-in-chief of the new Peter Bent Brigham Hospital in Boston.

Long afterward, Cushing stated that he considered it highly fortunate that the surgery on General Wood had been so successful, considering the positive attitude to the possibilities of brain surgery that developed after that very operation.

General Wood in the Period from 1910 to 1920

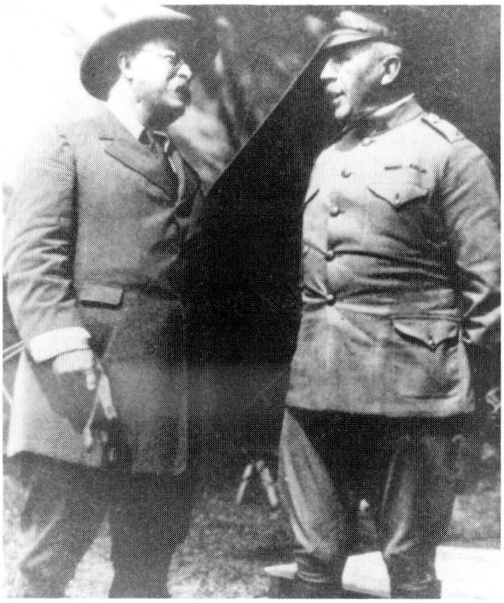

Figure 24: *Theodore Roosevelt (left) and General Wood at Plattsburg, New York, in 1915.*

During the following decade, Wood led an extremely active life (Fig 24). He had no epileptic seizures and felt himself to be completely healthy, with unimpaired vigor and in as good a condition as before the tumor symptoms appeared, except for moderate spasticity in the left foot, which apparently caused him no worry to speak of. There were many who were witness to his indefatigable energy and his predilection for strenous physical exertion. In this period he also published *The Military Obligations of Citizenship* (1915), *Our Military History, Its Facts and Fallacies* (1916), and *Universal Military Training* (1917).

Toward the end of World War I, when Wood was making an inspection tour of the front in France, a shell burst in his immediate vicinity, killing several of those standing nearby. Wood himself was severely wounded, as were two of his adjutants. Wood was the only one of the survivors to show no sign of what was called "shell shock." He quickly recovered, and his energy remained as unflagging as ever.

In that same year, he underwent a thorough medical checkup before a medical commission in Washington. At one point he was required to hop around on one leg; one of the examining surgeons remarked, "He maybe doesn't hop quite the way I would hop—but God Almighty, he sure can hop!" The entire commission of expert physicians were unanimous in their conclusion: never had they seen such a splendid specimen of health and strength as General Wood.

The Intrigues Around the Post-Wilson Presidency

In the 1920 presidential election campaign, Wood, the personification of competence, became the Republican favorite. Harry Daugherty, a rather odd gentleman and lawyer, who liked to busy himself in what came to be known as "the smoke-filled room of American politics" was, however, to cause a totally unexpected outcome of the presidential campaign.

For years Daugherty had been working away on the quiet to bring to the presidency a man who would serve his own interests: Warren Gamaliel Harding, editor in chief of a small country newspaper. Harding was willing to give lunchtime speeches, and the Republican Party often made use of him as a representative figure, but he had no ambition whatsoever of a big-time political career. Daugherty, however, got him elected to the Senate. When the nominating convention met in Chicago in August 1920, none of the ballots gave either Leonard Wood or his Republican competitor a sufficient majority; Senator Harding was launched as a third man for nomination, and subsequently was elected as president.

General Wood in the Period from 1920 to 1927

After he had been eliminated from the presidential election campaign, Wood was appointed governor of the Philippines. While he was there—in the next year—he began to suffer sporadic seizures, with spasms in the left foot. Wood paid little attention to these warning signs, pursuing his duties at the same fast tempo as always. By 1923, the spasticity in the left leg had increased, and now partial paralysis of the arm set in too. Wood, however, still took part in shooting competitions, with a surer aim than most of his fellow competitors, even with his left arm!

In April 1927, Wood was involved in a car accident. He was thrown out of the car, suffering a severe trauma to the right side of the head. Even before this accident, he had had a fairly pronounced hemiparesis, although this had not prevented him from conscientiously carrying out all his duties as governor.

He used the accident as a justification for terminating his governorship, and returned to the United States, where he submitted an official report to President Coolidge. Only after this did he seek help from a specialist for his sickness. He was immediately admitted to the Peter Bent Brigham Hospital where Cushing had been senior physician since 1912.

When he came under Cushing's care on August 4, 1927, Wood had a severe spastic hemiparesis on the left side, with contractures also in the arm, and a pronounced central facial paresis. With considerable difficulty he was able to get up from a chair, stand, and take a few stumbling steps with someone to support him. He also had a complete homonymous hemianopia and otherwise such severely reduced vision that he was unable to read ordinary printed text.

General Wood's Last Operation

Cushing, who was now at the height of his career, had just returned from Britain, where in the course of a single month he had been awarded no less than seven distinctions from different medical societies. Deeply concerned at Wood's condition, he decided to operate on the tumor recurrence as soon as possible.

The operation was performed only two days later, on August 6, 1927; it revealed a very large tumor. Cushing, who had started surgery in the morning, suggested after many hours that the completion of the tumor removal should be postponed. However, Wood begged to have it over with. From time to time, Wood talked to Cushing, even cracking a joke and occasionally saying he was doing well and hoped others were the same! There was loss of blood and twice blood was transfused from medical students.

Finally, Cushing was able to complete the extirpation without any major complications during the long operation. Nonetheless, Wood died only a few hours after the operation was concluded of an unexpected hemorrhage that broke through into the ventricular system.

No tragedy caused Cushing more distress than the death of Wood. He could not bring himself to operate again for several weeks. He slept wretchedly, and told of how he lay awake every night for a week after the operation going over and over in his mind every step and reproaching himself for not having waited longer after his return from Europe before operating.

Cushing, in disappointment, noted, "On my return we were not yet in full swing. Nor were my surgical reflexes and judgment at their best. I've never lost a patient after operation that so upset me. It was so near to success. He was a great man." This was the reflection of another impressive personality, after operating on one who was a close friend and a famous public figure, who had almost been elected president of the United States.

Selected References

1. Cabot AT. Letter to Harvey Cushing, dated January 14, 1909. In: *Leonard Wood. 1860-1927. Harvey Cushing Collection.* New Haven, Connecticut: Yale Medical Historical Library.

2. Cushing H. The meningiomas (dural endotheliomas): their source, and favoured seats of origin. *Brain.* 1922;45:282-316.

3. Cushing H, Eisenhardt L. *Meningiomas: Their Classification, Regional Behavior, Life History, and Surgical End Results.* Springfield, Ill: Charles C Thomas Publisher; 1938:409-414.

4. Cushing H, Eisenhardt L. Notes on first reasonably successful removal of intracranial tumor. *Bull Los Angeles Neurol Soc.* 1938;3:95-98.

5. Durante F. Contribution to endocranial surgery. *Lancet.* 1887;2:654-655.

6. Durante F. Extirpazione di un tumore endocranico. *Bull Acad Med Roma.* 1885;11:247-252. Published in English in: *Buffalo Med Surg J.* 1885-1886;25:369.

7. Hagedorn H. *Leonard Wood. A Biography.* New York, NY: Harper and Brothers; 1931:(vol 1)1-436;(vol 2)1-524.

8. Holme JG. *The Life of Leonard Wood.* Garden City, NY: Doubleday-Page; 1920:1-228.

9. Jefferson G. Harvey Cushing April 8, 1869–October 7, 1939. *Surg Neurol.* 1974;2:217-224.

10. Keen WW. Three successful cases of cerebral surgery: including the removal of a large intracranial fibroma. *Am J Med Sci.* 1888;96:329-347.

11. Ljunggren B. The case of General Wood. *J Neurosurg.* 1982;56:471-474.

12. MacEwen W. Intracranial lesions. III: tumour of dura mater. Epileptic convulsions; trephining; removal of tumour from dura mater and orbital cavity; recovery. *Lancet.* 1882;1:40-44.

Chapter 6

Harvey Cushing and Sven Hedin

Sven Hedin (1865-1952) was a Swedish explorer of Asia who won a worldwide reputation for his many discoveries and immense series of publications. He formed friendships with many outstanding personalities of the first half of the 20th century, whom he described in a grand opus, *Great Men and Kings.* Among his best friends was Harvey Cushing. The warm friendship between the two giants is evident in their correspondence.

This chapter includes a brief description of Sven Hedin and his life's work, and how fate brought him to Boston in 1929.

At the age of 20, Hedin, four years older than his contemporary Harvey Cushing, rode through Persia with his student's cap at a jaunty angle. Fifty years later in Peking he completed his last expedition. In between lay his extensive expeditions through all of Central Asia.

Under tremendous hardship and grueling and hazardous conditions, he crossed territories that were at that time completely unknown to Westerners. He forced the tableland of Pamir and nearly perished in the Takla Makan desert. He solved the mystery of Lop-nor, "the wandering lake," and mapped unknown parts of the huge massif, which he named Transhimalaya. He spent one New Year's Eve with the Holy Tashi Lama (Fig 25); he discovered the springs of the Indus and Brahmaputra, and found the remains of Lou-lan, the wondrous city that had lain buried and forgotten in the desert for more than 1,000 years by the time Marco Polo made his famous expedition through Asia in 1274. While excavating in Lou-lan, Hedin found what were then the oldest specimens of paper* containing written characters known in the world, as well as pieces of bamboo with written characters on them dating back 1,800 years.

Hedin, who was warm-hearted, somewhat naive, and unaware of the bestiality of people such as Adolf Hitler, was sometimes misled when involved with top-level politics. He got along well with emperors and great celebrities as well as with the more primitive Asian companions on his expeditions, and it is well documented that he showed the same warm amiability to all people.

All that he undertook assumed extreme dimensions: the heights of the mountains he climbed, the depths of the deserts he crossed, the distances of his excursions, the number of works he published, and the many marks of distinction he acquired during his career.†

Hedin's *Central Asia Atlas*, covering the vast territories that he, his chief geologist Erik Norin, and his paleontologist Birger Bohlin (who in 1927 confirmed the existence of Homo pekinensis) explored by camel in the 1920s and 1930s, was published during the years 1952-1959. During the past 15 years, the mapping of the earth by the U.S. National Aeronautics and Space Administration, using the Earth Resources Test Satellite system, has shown Hedin's atlas to be essentially correct.

In 1947, at the age of 82 and practically blind, Hedin, despite all other obligations, began to write a new grand opus, *Great Men and Kings*, a two-volume work of more than 1,000 pages in which he describes 61 men and two women. Completed and published in

*Paper was invented by a eunuch at the Chinese emperor's court by the year A.D. 105. It was not until the 11th century that the art of making paper was brought to Europe. The documents from Lou-lan were later deciphered by a German professor, Conrady, in Leipzig.

†Among all Hedin's honors, his honorary doctorates at Oxford and Cambridge Universities, announced within three days of each other in March 1909, and his nomination to Knight Commander of the Indian Empire, implying the possession of a British peerage, need to be mentioned.

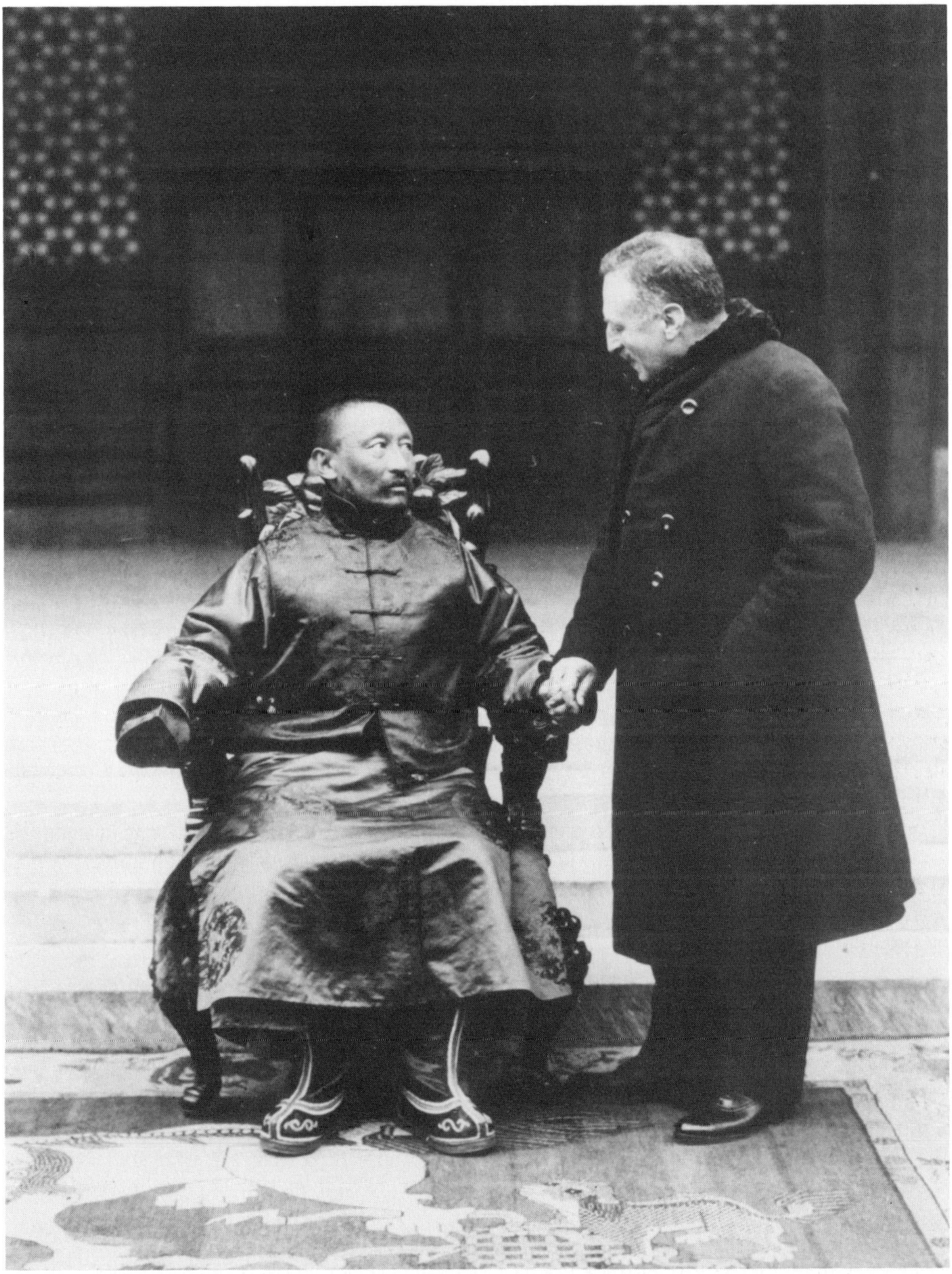

Figure 25: *Sven Hedin at an audience with the reincarnated Tashi Lama, "The Holy Teacher," in Shigatse. The Dalai Lama, "The Holy King," in Lhasa was at this time (beginning of 1907) in exile. The Holy Lama showered valuable gifts on Hedin, who repaid him by offering the Lama the contents in his Burroughs Wellcome pharmaceutical box.*

1950, this work is a gold mine for those who wish to learn more about distant parts of the world, significant events, and fascinating personalities of the first half of this century.

In *Great Men and Kings*, Hedin describes the following people: two women—the Swedish Queen Victoria and the famous authoress Selma Lagerlöf; the kaisers Franz Josef and Wilhelm II; the emperor of Japan, Mutsuhito, and the emperor of Korea, Lee Chouk; the Russian czar, Nicolai II; the shah of Persia, Nasr-ed-Din; the sultan of Turkey, Abdul Hamid II; King Boris of Bulgaria and several other kings; Lord Kitchener of Khartoum and Lord Curzon; the generals Nogi, Baden-Powell, von Hindenburg, and Ludendorff; the field marshals von Mackensen and Mannerheim of Finland; Sir Henry Morton Stanley and the arctic explorers Nordenskiöld, Andrée, Nansen, Amundsen, and Scott; Pope Pius X, Chiang Kai-shek, Alfred Nobel; and finally the Americans—Theodore Roosevelt, Henry Ford, and Harvey Cushing.

When Hedin died in 1952 at the age of 88, 32 volumes of his *Reports from the Scientific Expedition* had been published. The number had reached 54 by 1977 and at that time constituted, apart from maps and pictures, about 20,000 pages.

Over the course of 65 years, Hedin published an outstanding series of geographical accounts covering his many expeditions, biographies, and autobiographies, and an immense and incalculable number of minor publications on geographical, political, and general topics.

In addition, the Sven Hedin Archives in Stockholm comprises 80,000 letters, reflecting the fact that he always made it a point of honor to reply personally to all letters. The archives of Sven Hedin, fully accessible since 1977 for research purposes, mirror the range of the world's events—from the great discoveries made in the 19th century through the period of optimism accompanying the rapid developments at the turn of the century into the revolutionary events of the present epoch.

Hedin's Meeting with Cushing

On February 2, 1929, Hedin woke in the middle of the night with a terrible pain in his right shoulder. Dr. Dick Hummel,* the physician who accompanied Hedin everywhere on his Asian excursions, was consulted and Hedin was transferred to the Peking Union Medical College (P.U.M.C.) of the Rockefeller Foundation. He was treated there by a "staff of specialists from many countries and within some weeks the pain was gone." Accompanied by Hummel, Hedin left on February 25th for Nanking, where he was to meet with Chiang Kai-shek.

On April 24, he was "struck by a violent relapse and was again admitted to P.U.M.C." It was then believed that Hedin suffered from a cervical spinal tumor and that he should immediately be referred to Harvey Cushing in Boston. A visiting Swedish professor at the P.U.M.C. telegraphed Cushing, who answered that Hedin was welcome to come to Boston.

On May 21, 1929, Hedin, accompanied by Hummel, left China aboard the steamship President Taft bound for Yokohama. Via Victoria, they reached Seattle on June 3 and then

*Hummel was in fact consulted by the noble and the poor—those dying of phthisis, those infected by syphilis, those with eye diseases, and those unfortunates addicted to opium—and his "wonder" cures had strengthened the reputation of the expedition in many sensitive situations.

traveled by the train The Olympian to Chicago. On June 8, they arrived in Buffalo, where Hedin met his sister Alma and Professor Einar Key from Stockholm, who was in the United States to attend a surgical convention. Key examined Hedin and became skeptical of the diagnosis made by the doctors in Peking, but nevertheless recommended that Hedin be examined by Cushing.

At the Peter Bent Brigham Hospital, Hedin "got a room and was subjected to a cross-examination of Cushing's assistant, Dr. Scarff," who in his turn was cross-examined concerning the abilities of Cushing, "the man that now had my fate in his hand." According to Hedin, Scarff described Cushing as a charming man who performed his operations with great calm and with admirable safety.

The two giants first met on June 11 (Fig 26). As Hedin described the meeting, the door opened and in came "a thin and wiry, distinguished gentleman with light brown, vivacious, intelligent and jovial eyes. He had an aquiline nose, shortcut hair, was stylish and noble, greeting me gaily and kindly as if we had been acquainted with each other since childhood. Within a moment, a bond of friendship was bound with Harvey Cushing, which was to last and only grow stronger until the day a decade later when he, on the threshold of the Second World War, went to his final rest."

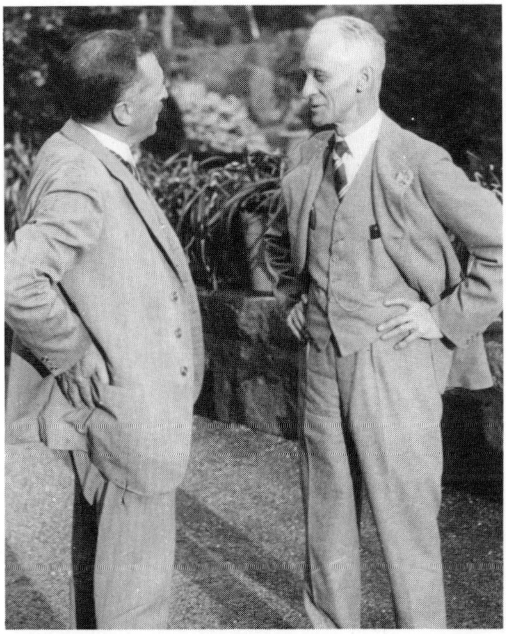

Figure 26: *Sven Hedin and Harvey Cushing in Boston in 1929. (Photograph by Dick Hummel.)*

After the examination, Cushing assured Hedin that he found no evidence of a tumor. Alma, his sister, was also told the good news and "there was general happiness." Hedin then asked Cushing:

"How shall I now behave?"

"You shall stay here for another 10 days."

"For observation?"

"No, to give me the opportunity to show you all subjects, views, and monuments of interest in Boston and to introduce you to some interesting American families, descendants of the Mayflower immigrants settling on Cape Cod in the year of 1620."

"And then?"

"Then you return after some time to your expedition in Sinkiang if you haven't had a relapse within that time!"

"Splendid! Your diagnosis, Dr. Cushing, is worth such a journey and it would be worth the trouble to go around the world many times to get acquainted with you!" was Hedin's reply.

Over the next few days, Cushing took his patient on many unforgettable excursions, including the Commencement Day exercises at Harvard University at which Franklin D. Roosevelt was presented with an honorary doctorate. A visit was paid to the famous Saturday Club, where Hedin was introduced to the president of Harvard University, Dr. Lowell, and to Jeremias Smith, who had just arrived from the Young conference in Paris.

Meanwhile Hummel and Dr. René Leriche, who was visiting at the same time, observed some of Cushing's operations. And to the P.U.M.C. Cushing telegraphed, "No further trouble. No indication for surgery." On June 22, Einar Key arrived in Boston and he and Cushing performed a second examination. It again revealed normal findings, and the next day Hedin left Boston and his new friend.

Hedin was in urgent need of more money for his next expedition and traveled back to Chicago to see a rich industrialist of Swedish descent, Vincent Bendix, who owned the Bendix Brake Company. Bendix had run away from home and started his career as an elevator attendant at the age of 16. He by then was living in a magnificent private villa with 75 rooms and was "a man who enjoyed life to the full." Bendix told Hedin that he had for a long time been considering doing something for his old country. Hedin mentioned that he had recently received half a million from the Swedish king.

"Then I will give you the same amount," Bendix answered, then asked, "Was it half a million dollars or crowns?"

"Crowns," Hedin answered truthfully.

Much later, Hedin was asked if there was anything he regretted doing in his life. "Perhaps that I didn't say 'dollars' instead of 'crowns' to Mr. Bendix. It would have made no difference to him. Shortly afterward his whole empire went to rack and ruin in the global depression."

With a clean bill of health and new funds, Hedin returned in high spirits and without symptoms to Stockholm, where he immediately started the final preparations for his next expedition. He noted that "the pain had appeared because one night I sat at a drafty window in Peking. I froze but had no time to go to bed because I had to finish a report that had to be handed over to the China Committee the following morning." Cushing had found it "remarkable that the severe shoulder pain had both times appeared very acutely and then slowly disappeared."

Hedin and Cushing's Friendship

As a result of Hedin's acquaintance with Cushing, Cushing was soon invited to visit Sweden. In early autumn of the same year, Cushing repaid Hedin's visit to Boston by including a trip to Sweden as part of a journey to Europe (Fig 27). The six days spent in Sweden, Cushing's only visit to that country, have been thoroughly described in Fulton's biography.

It was during those hectic days that Cushing coined the word Hummelism—for Hummel's relentless efforts to stretch the short time Cushing had available for the visit. There were so many libraries, scientific collections, and hospitals to look at and prominent people to meet that Hummel had to stick to a rigid timetable. The prominent guest was not allowed to exceed the schedule by more than five minutes!

At the end of his visit, Cushing proposed that an "Antihummelism Society" should be founded! The great American was also introduced to the Swedish King Gustaf V, who jocularly asked Cushing how in fact things were with Sven Hedin.

Cushing also had been invited to Lund by the young Swedish pathologist Arvid Lindau, who two years earlier had described the cerebellar hemangioma. On September 4, at the Medical Society in Lund, Cushing lectured on the medulloblastomas, a talk that was well received. Afterward, a grand dinner was given by the medical faculty of the university. The

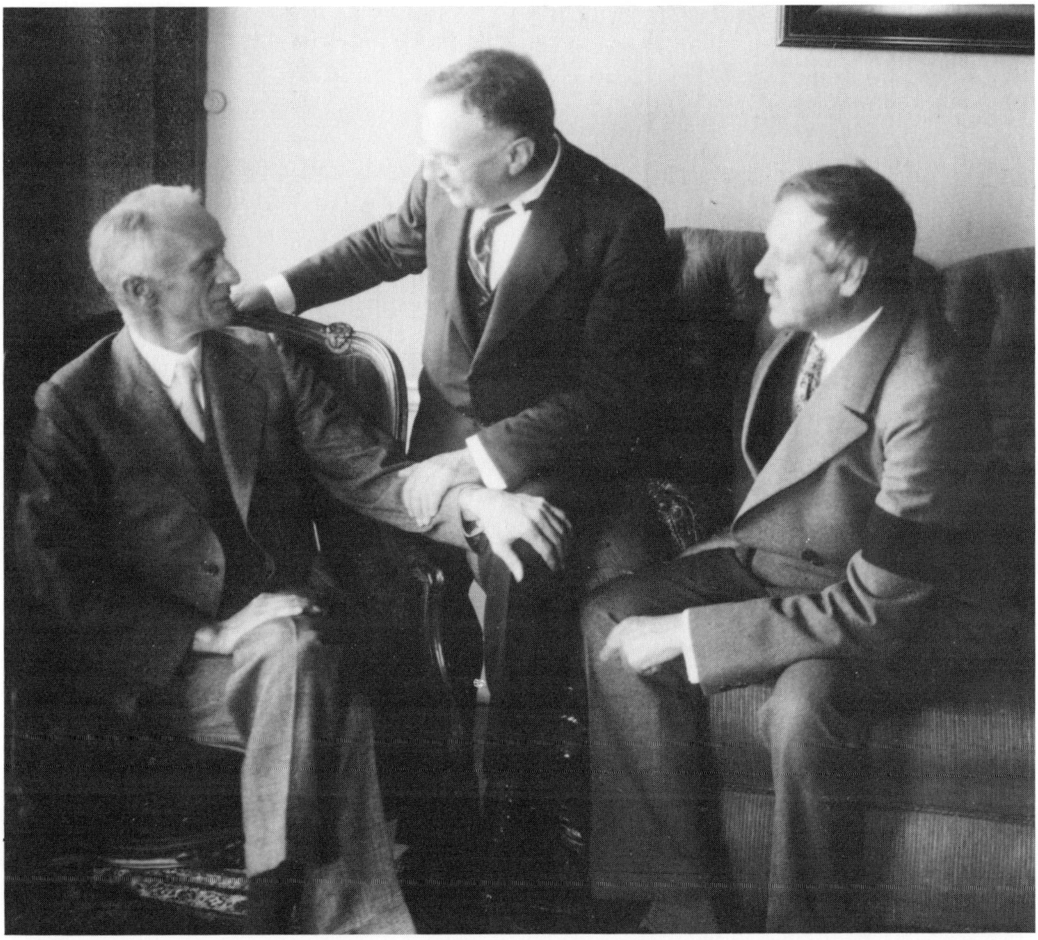

Figure 27: *Harvey Cushing at Sven Hedin's home in Stockholm, September, 1929. From left to right: Cushing, Hedin, and Einar Key, professor of surgery in Stockholm.*

medical students and the doctors were seated in the large hall of the Academic Club, while Cushing was seated with the most prominent professors and local celebrities in a smaller adjacent room. After coffee, Cushing got up and joined the students and younger doctors in the large hall.

At this time, he happened to talk with a young doctor, Åke Rydén, who was an old friend of Hummel's and had corresponded for some time with Hummel concerning Hedin's symptoms. Rydén, whose main interest at that time concerned brachial neuralgia and other neuralgiform pains, had informed Hummel that, in his opinion, Hedin most probably did not suffer from a spinal cord tumor. He told Cushing about his ideas concerning the diagnosis. Cushing was amused and told Rydén that he was absolutely right. Hedin's trip to Boston had been unnecessary but, on the other hand, was very rewarding since it had resulted in Cushing's invitation to visit Sweden and the opportunity to make so many new acquaintances. Cushing then circulated among the tables and apparently enjoyed speaking with the younger colleagues.

At the Royal Library in Stockholm, Cushing became especially interested in a three-meter-long parchment roll containing depictions of human diseases and their treatment that was hand drawn and colored—a scientific work of art by John of Ardene that had been presented to the king of Pomerania as a gift from his wife, Queen Filippa, in the early 15th century.

After Cushing's departure, Hedin ordered the Generalstabens Litografiska Anstalt* in Stockholm to make a copy "so true to the original that only an expert could determine which was the original and which was the copy." Even faults and stains were strictly copied. The parchment roll had the title: "Practica Magistri Johannis Ardeni de Newark; De arte phisical & de Cirurgia 1412." There are two vertical columns with Latin text placed between three files of 118 illustrations. It took some months to complete the copy.

Cushing was delighted to receive the gift. After his return to Boston he wrote to Alma Hedin on December 19, 1929:

"The copy of that precious Ardene MS has come safely through the kind intermediation of the Consul-General in New York. I cannot possibly tell you how thrilled and excited I am to possess it. It is truly a marvellous facsimile. I can hardly imagine how it could have been so perfectly done. It will make the most precious item in my medico-historical collection. I shall write to Sven to express my great appreciation. It is so like him to have thought of it. I would much rather have it than a lama temple.† I hope you are having good news from the expedition and I trust that the disorders in Manchuria have not in any way affected Mongolia. But then, Sven has a charmed life and with Hummel to keep an eye on him and to see that he stays on the shady side of his dromedary, we may all feel he is quite safe."

And to Sven Hedin, Cushing wrote the following:

"That marvellous copy of the Ardene MS that you have had made for me in celebration, I presume, of the operation I did not perform on your spinal marrow has come just in time for Christmas. And such a present!

It is an absolutely perfect facsimile of the original—indeed, I am not quite sure but that they have made a mistake and sent me the original. But I will keep mum about this. I will also keep mum about the fact that Hummel and not I really deserved this reward. For it was he that turned the trick and cured you en route to America and not I.

Words fail me to tell you what store I set upon this MS, which will always remain far the most precious item in my library—doubly precious not only in its intrinsic value but because of its association for me with you and your sisters.

By this time, I suppose you are undulating in that favourite position of yours, ensconced between the humps of a dromedary while you are writing your notes and sketching the wonders of creation (Fig 28).

I hope you will be able to find and select the lama temples without great delay and difficulty, so that you can devote yourself to the geographical problems that interest you far more than these ethnological matters interest you. Still, so far as I can gather, nothing exists that fails to interest you. You are not one of those people who have what we call a single-track mind.

---

*The same engraving establishment that printed all Hedin's Asian maps.

†Hedin had promised Bendix a complete genuine lama temple in return for the half million crowns Bendix had donated to Hedin's expedition.

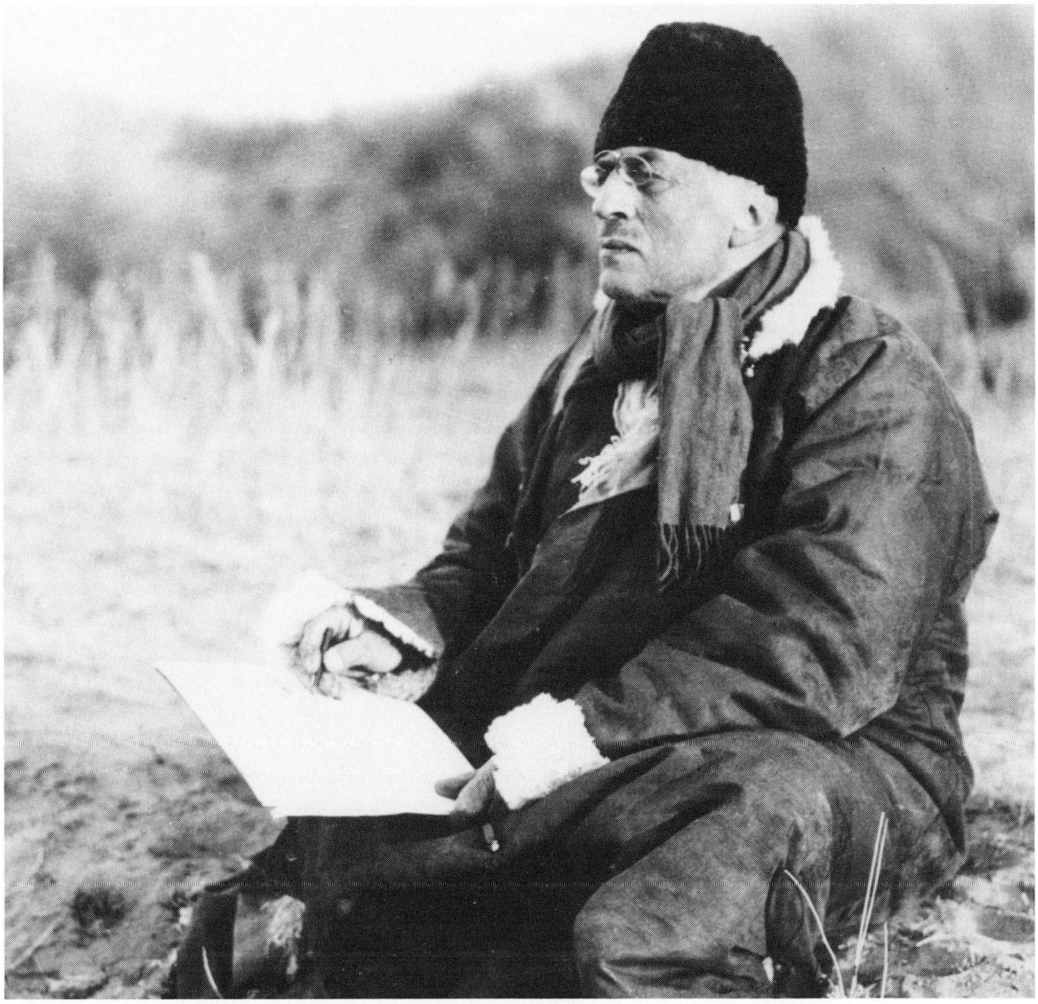

Figure 28: *Sven Hedin was, like Harvey Cushing, an excellent artist. Here he is seen sketching the landscape somewhere in Asia.*

If you or Dick should run across any old Mongolian or Tibetan medical MSS which contain diagrams with the Oriental conception of anatomy, I hope you will beg, buy, or steal them for my collection. I have a few Persian and Arabic MSS and I would like to compare the figures in them with the figures which occur in the older Chinese MSS where I suppose one must find the originals that perhaps were the source-books of the kind.

We shall have fun together when we next meet but I shall never expect to have a better time than we had during the hectic week in Sweden, when we were all so Hummelised."

By November 1929, Hedin had already returned to a small monastery town in inner Mongolia, and from there his expedition started: "And as small dots the camel columns disappeared against the endless plains of the Gobi Desert for a ride that should come to extend over a distance of 1,112 kilometers."

On February 17, 1931, Cushing wrote to Alma Hedin:

"You will be sorry to learn that I am laid up in the hospital and I think I had better send for Hummel. They are making an awful lot of fuss over me, over very little, so far as I can see.

And now for something much more important: namely, a long thrilling and most enthusiastic letter from Sven telling about the success of his many expeditions and about Dick Hummel's safe return after having been captured more times by bandits than you have sisters. . . .

That the Chinese officials finally have succumbed to him is no surprise to me. The only matter of surprise is that they should have been able to resist as long as they did. I suppose that he will now be sitting up 'til 6:00 A.M. writing some of these things down with his usual industry and smoking innumerable cigarettes; and the only thing I want to warn you about is not to let him do so before an open window with a Swedish north wind blowing on his back.

You can please tell that man Hummel that I only think of him once a day and that is when I take my morning shave. But as for the rest of you, I think of you continuously. I hope this will make him feel very bad because, after all, I never have been quite the same man since he had me on that five-minute schedule."

In February 1932, Hedin returned to America to set up the lama temple for Bendix as he had promised. On his way to Chicago he stayed three days in Boston with Cushing. As he later recalled, "We would sit the entire evening far into the night looking at his dear collection of manuscripts and aged leather volumes. One morning he woke me up earlier than usual. He held the morning paper in his hand and was very upset after having read that Charles Lindbergh's small son had been kidnapped the previous evening. He walked disturbed to and fro in the room explaining that no punishment could be hard enough for such villainy."

In Chicago, Hedin stayed as Bendix's guest in Potter Palmer's house on Michigan Avenue. In the huge gallery of that house was arranged a magnificent collection of Asian artifacts that would later be housed in the lama temple. While in Chicago, Hedin started the writing of a new book, *Conquest of Tibet.* The bed in his sleeping room was a magnificent piece of furniture. He described it, "Its immense canopy was supported by four screwn columns; at the gablefield a painting representing Darius at the battle of Issos was mounted and here and there cupids and ornaments could be seen." Bendix declared that the future king of England, George VI, on a visit to Chicago had slept in this royal parade bed.

One day early in the summer of 1932, Cushing, accompanied by two younger doctors, visited Hedin in Chicago, and he showed them the historical bed. By Hedin's account, Cushing, who rarely missed the opportunity for a good joke, turned to his colleagues and with sepulchral gravity said, "This is Dr. Hedin's camp-bed. He has brought it with him on all his Asian journeys." According to Hedin, the two doctors looked at Cushing with astonishment and then at Hedin. "In reality, four Indian elephants would have been demanded to carry the huge and clumsy creature!"

On September 1, 1933, Cushing wrote to Hedin:

"I have been driven from pillar to post all summer and have been living alone in another world—namely, in a little back laboratory room in the Brigham Hospital trying to complete some neglected work before we move to New Haven. This will be about the time you will be moving westward on your new expedition. I do hope this letter and one

from the President will reach you before you start. He will be simply delighted with the stamps, I am sure.*

I am ashamed of myself for neglecting your letter so long, but it is only one, I grieve to say, of many that I have somehow not managed to answer. In spite of all your colossal work, you never allow your personal correspondence to suffer, and I know that an additional letter goes every day to your beloved sisters. All this shames me the more for my neglect to you, but when I get immersed in a task I promptly lose contact with everything else—family and friends included.

I saw in the papers that you are going off on this expedition for the Chinese Government and that it will be all that you desire as a culminating experience to your 48 (!) years in Asia.

Thanks to the new administration and Mr. Roosevelt, things are distinctly looking up in this country and I think this is being reflected everywhere in spite of the uneasiness Europe is feeling in regard to Hitler and his program. But the Germans are too solid a people to be wholly and permanently carried away by his military ambitions.

Take good care of yourself, my dear friend. I'm so glad Dick is to accompany you, and I wish I might go as supercargo, so that I could be with you both. But the thought of 20 consecutive days on a camel makes me uncertain. I'm not well upholstered for that."

In February 1934, Cushing wrote to Alma:

"When I think of Sven sleeping in a tent with below zero temperature in the center of Asia, surrounded by bandits and Lord knows what else, it makes me feel a perfect good-for-nothing. Still, I suppose that even I might make a go of it with Hummel to tie me up in my sleeping bag every night and pat me on the back.

I am so happy to learn from your letter, just come, of my having been made a member of the Swedish Academy of Sciences. It is truly a great honor."

In another letter to Alma, June 16, 1934, he wrote the following:

"Thanks hugely for sending me the interesting photographs of the Mongolian medical plates. They are just the sort of thing that interest me greatly. I have seen Persian medical plates allied to these Mongolian plates, and the development of this early crude anatomy in those Eastern countries is a very interesting part of medical history. I shall have them bound and put in my library with your note about them."

On March 26, 1935, he wrote to Alma:

"So happy to have the good news that Sven is celebrating his 70th birthday safe and sound at Nanking and that his sisters will expect to see him at home within a month. What a time of hardship and difficulties to overcome this expedition must have been! I suppose no one will ever really know all that he has been through, what with bandits, typhoid fever, shivering for weeks in a skimping tent. What a Stoic he is!

I have known other people just like that—not too many, to be sure—who waive aside all the disagreeable things of life as though they never existed and plow through all obstacles between them and their goal with head up and a smile on their face. I suppose it is the spirit of all great explorers, and we who sit at home comfortably and spend our time avoiding the risks they so cheerfully take can but marvel at it. I must send him a cable of welcome and will try the Swedish Embassy, but suppose Sven Hedin, Asia, would be enough."

---

*Hedin's expedition had been awarded the rare privilege of a Chinese issue of a series of stamps depicting a halting place in Mongolia, showing a caravan of camels and the pennant of the expedition. Hedin had sent a first-day issue to Franklin D. Roosevelt, who was a stamp collector.

At this time Hummel, who was collecting insects as well as serving as physician to Hedin, had published his first two descriptive volumes on insects, and he presented copies to Cushing. In a letter to Alma, Cushing wrote the following:

"And then Dick has actually had the effrontery to name a particular atrocious bug after Sven in which 'Die Unterschiede sind folgende: Scheitel mitten etwas gewölbter, Gesicht nach unten etwas weniger verschmälert, Punktierung des Scheitels etwas stärker und dichter,' etc. (The characteristics are as follows: crown somewhat vaulted in the middle, face narrowing slightly from top to bottom, peak of the head fairly strong and compact.) I don't dare look any further because I may find something still worse named after me. It would be just like him to have gotten back at me in this way with a scientific camouflage after (my) making fun of his Hummelism."

On October 20, 1936, Cushing gave his thanks for having received Hedin's latest publication, *The Flight of Big Horse*, and wrote the following:

"When some day in the remote future you go to Valhalla reserved for all famous explorers, the first person to greet you, I am sure, will be Marco Polo, and what a pow-wow you will have together!

We are here in the thick of the political campaign and in our house naturally hope that the president will be reelected. When next you come over here and he is still in the White House, we will go and pay him a visit together."

Cushing wrote the following in his customary Christmas letter, sent December 1937:

"It all goes to show what a wonderful race you are and what a good example your friend the king, now almost an octogenarian, sets for you.

But then, both Sven and I will be octogenarians before we know it and I would like to apply for a room near his where we might share a common barrel of ink on the roof with one tube leading to his pen and another to mine. Or one pipe might do for both of us as he is a nocturnal and I a diurnal scribbler. Or if we grow tired of that, he can make sketches and I will take up embroidery, for I used to be a fairly good stitcher—at least on the skin."

Hedin had hoped that Cushing would visit him in Stockholm in the spring of 1938, but the journey did not come about. Cushing wrote to Hedin blaming "that Hummelism business which makes life so arduous, for I am not so athletic as I once was."

In a letter of April 12, in which Cushing described the celebration of his 70th birthday, he wrote the following:

"A handsomely bound volume containing a collection of papers written by my Scandinavian doctor friends and printed in Acta Chirurgica Scandinavica* *was presented to me at the dinner by young Olof Sjöquist who made a gracious speech. I looked through the volume eagerly thinking you might have contributed something of personal experiences with pseudo-tumors of the spinal cord."*

On October 7, 1939, Hedin had dinner with some good friends at his home in Stockholm. The guests had been welcomed and one of them, Dr. Giertz, reminded those assembled that he had participated at the dinner given almost a decade earlier for Cushing. Hence the topic of conversation happened to be the great American. While the guests were still seated at the dinner table, a telegram arrived with these few words:

New Haven, Hedin, Stockholm. Harvey died quietly this morning. Kate.

---

*The initiative for the publication, which was dedicated to Cushing, had been taken by Erik Ask-Upmark, professor of internal medicine in Uppsala, Sweden, who had come to Boston to study Cushing's unique archives of brain tumors some months after Cushing's retirement in 1932.

Hedin commented later:
"It was as though the light had gone out and a deep shadow come over us. He had stood out not only as the unrivaled doctor, but first of all a man of exceptionally great dimensions, a chieftain amongst the elite of guests on earth. In my memory I shall preserve and bless him as the most outstanding, the most noble and most beloved of great men that I have met during my way through life.

Had his heart broken by the thought of a new world war between those human beings, who he had always wanted to help and cure? He had had more than enough of the first World War and did not stand another."

Surprising Autopsy Findings

The autopsy of Harvey Cushing revealed multiple old cerebral infarcts and also many scattered glial scars. One pial artery in the right motor area was found completely occluded by an organized thrombus. This vessel as well as numerous others of arterial and arteriolar size in the meninges and brain parenchyma showed pronounced atheromatous changes. In fact, Cushing had himself surmised that paraesthesias and weakness of the fingers of his left hand were caused by a focal cortical lesion. The autopsy certainly revealed how accurate his diagnosis had been. Furthermore, there was a slight degree of internal hydrocephalus affecting both lateral ventricles as the result of a gray, fleshy, spherical cyst filled with a homogeneous colloid and hanging from the tela chorioidea of the third ventricle.

Harry Zimmerman, who performed the autopsy, incorrectly attributed Cushing's disease from 1918 to occlusion of the abdominal aorta. Cushing dated the onset of this illness to August 6, 1918: "this was the beginning of my encephalo-polyneuritis from which I was nearly two years in recovering and then incompletely."

Cushing's biographer, John Fulton, mistakenly labeled the illness a "vascular polyneuritis." Today, this one of Cushing's illnesses is recognized as Guillain-Barré syndrome.

In the case of Cushing's friend Hedin, who was to survive him by 13 years, the autopsy findings (regarding Hedin) were even more surprising and interesting. Quite unexpectedly it was revealed that the sella turcica was filled with an upwards bulging homogeneous cyst. One may speculate to which extent this pituitary cystic adenoma had influenced the life of the great explorer. Maybe a decrease in pituitary function already in younger years was the true explanation why Hedin had preferred to devote his life to exploration of Central Asia instead of the female sex!

One may but conclude that Cushing and Hedin were *great men* with major achievements during life. Yet in both cases autopsy revealed that they had *sick brains.*

Selected References

1. Brenneke D. *Sven Hedin.* Hamburg, Germany: Rowohlt Taschenbuch Verlag, GmbH; 1986.

2. Fulton JF. *Harvey Cushing. A Biography.* Springfield, Ill: Charles C Thomas Publisher; 1946.

3. Kaneko T. *Hedin-den. Idai-na shirukurodo no tankensha.* Tokyo, Japan: Publishing Co; 1980.

4. Kish G. *To the Heart of Asia: The Life of Sven Hedin.* Ann Arbor, Mich: The University of Michigan Press; 1984.

5. Ljunggren B. Harvey Cushing and Sven Hedin. *Surgical Neurology.* 1982;17:165-171.

6. Reich SG. Harvey Cushing's Guillain-Barré Syndrome: An historical diagnosis. *Neurosurgery.* 1987;21:135-141.

7. Wennerholm E. *Sven Hedin. A Biography.* Stockholm, Sweden: Bonniers; 1978.

8. Zimmerman HM. The last days of Harvey Cushing. *Surg Neurol.* 1975;3:163-170.

Chapter 7

The Case of George Gershwin

The Prussian invasion of France and the unification of Germany in 1870 spurred Czar Alexander II to reform the Russian army, in which he took a strong interest. A St. Petersburg gunsmith, Gershovitz, reported that he had invented a new automatic weapon, which Alexander II much admired and for which the czar bought the rights from the inventor. Gershovitz was doubly happy as his wife had given birth to a son, Morris, in early 1871.

In 1891, a well-to-do Russian furrier by the name of Bruskin left St. Petersburg and emigrated to the United States with his family. Morris Gershovitz followed in their tracks. He was not particularly attracted by the opportunities of the New World, but had fallen deeply in love with the teenage daughter of the Bruskin family, a lovely girl with intense eyes and soft, beautiful features. The Bruskins, like so many other immigrants, settled in the East Side of New York. Morris shortened his name to Gershvin, obtained well-paid employment, and lost no time in wooing and winning Rose Bruskin, marrying her in 1895.

The young Gershvin couple took up residence in a simple apartment over a pawnbroker's shop in New York. Just over a year later, their first child was born; his given name was Israel, but he was always known as Ira. The family soon moved to a larger apartment, where on September 26, 1898, another son was born. He was given the name of Jacob, but was always known as George. Later, when George began his professional career in the musical world, he changed the spelling of his surname to Gershwin, and the rest of the family followed his example.

The father's view of life was somewhat quixotic. Most of the time, although by no means always, the family was well off. For a while, Morris Gershwin owned and operated a chain of restaurants, at another time he was in charge of a number of bath houses, and later he devoted himself to the confectionery and coffee shop business, owning and running a chain of bakeries. For a time he busied himself with bookmaking, but from a financial point of view, this was a near disaster. During another period, the hotel he was running in Spring Valley looked likely to fail because he took in so many nonpaying friends and relatives.

George looked up to his father; the father seemed to have appreciated his son's talent, although when the tone poem *An American in Paris* was given its premiere by the New York Philharmonic Orchestra in December 1928, he did remark, "This is great music—it takes more than 20 minutes to get through the piece!" In 1924, Gershwin presented his *Rhapsody in Blue*. When in 1931 his father learned that George was pondering possible titles for what came to be known as his *Second Rhapsody*, he advised his son with complete gravity, "Call it Rhapsody in Blue No. 2, George, then you can go on and write Rhapsody in Blue No. 3, No. 4, and No. 5—you know, just like Beethoven."

In temperament, George took after his mother. He was obstinate, somewhat authoritarian, energetic, and restless. There had not been a single musically gifted person over several past generations of either the Bruskin or the Gershovitz family, and his parents were not particularly musical. Neither did George show any signs of musical talent in childhood. On the other hand, there was little in the home to encourage any musical interest. When George was 12, however, his mother brought a piano into the household. Within a few months, George was playing Sousa marches at the morning assemblies at school. At the age of 15, he was engaged as accompanist to a vocal group at a weekly salary of $15.

The Man They Loved

Gershwin's whole life soon became filled with his music. He liked nothing better than composing, playing, and talking music from morning until night (Fig 29). By disposition he was gentle, friendly, and generous toward people. He was as impassioned by his own music as by that of other popular composers such as Irving Berlin, Jerome Kern, and Hoagy Carmichael.

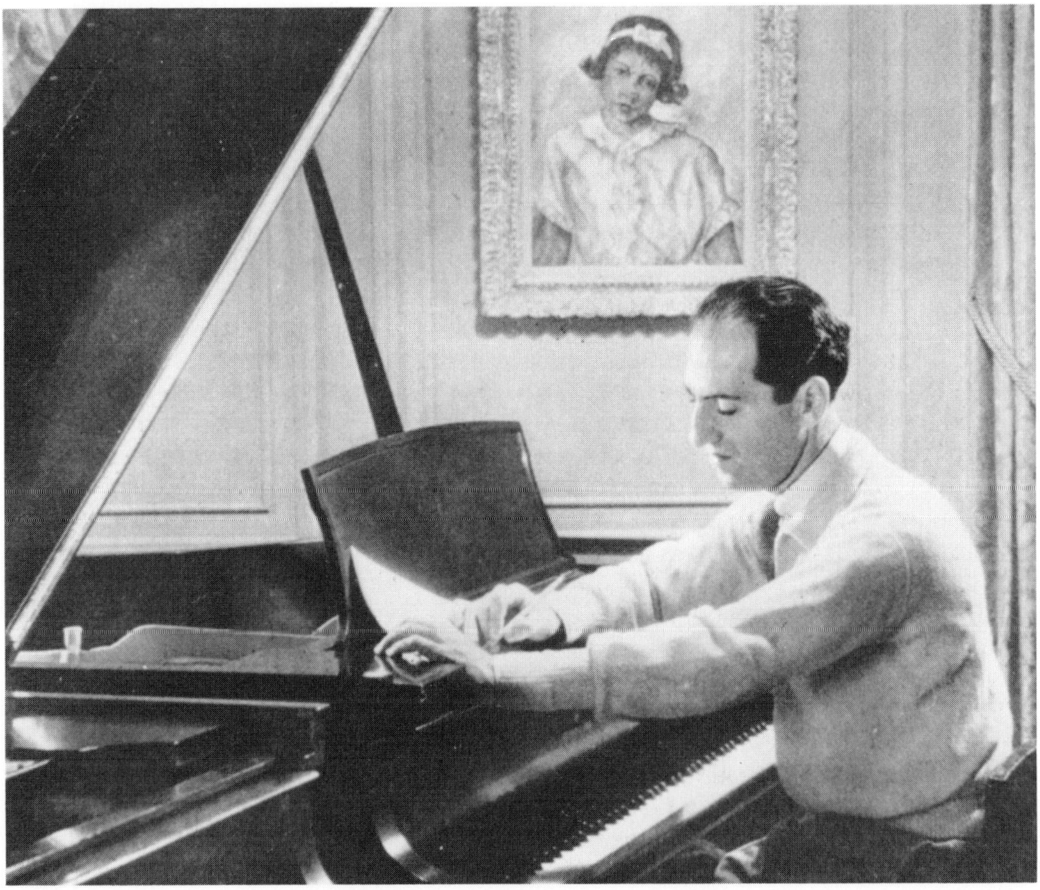

Figure 29: *George Gershwin at the piano.*

He was lively, and his walk almost always had a little skip to it whether he was in the street or on the golf course. He always went up stairs two at a time. When he was ill, his vitality was greater than that of most people in good health. He never lay idly abed even if he felt poorly. He possessed an irresistible enthusiasm and a voracious appetite for life.

A man of excellent physique, Gershwin would go in for any kind of sport: beside being a good golfer, an excellent horseman, and a competent swimmer, he could also enjoy a game of baseball. He was an accomplished dancer and could give a perfect imitation of Fred Astaire. At the dress rehearsal of *Lady Be Good,* he gave Fred Astaire valuable advice on how to dance the final steps in *Fascinating Rhythm.*

In 1928, Gershwin moved to a large studio apartment, which soon became a meeting place for the cream of New York theatre people, musicians, artists, and film actors. There were always people coming and going, and musical compositions were tried out and composed on Gershwin's large Steinway piano. The atmosphere has been described as resembling that of a large railway station.

In 1929, the sound film came, and soon the film magnates began to take notice of George's musical production. In 1932, he wrote his first film musical, *Girl Crazy*. In the autumn of 1933, Gershwin began to compose his most important work, the opera *Porgy and Bess*, which was to take him almost two years to complete. His musicals were enormously successful on Broadway and throughout the United States. In 1932, he was awarded the Pulitzer Prize. In 1935, with his brother Ira, Gershwin moved to Hollywood, there to rent what was in effect a small palace with a swimming pool and its own tennis courts in Beverly Hills; the place soon attracted the top Hollywood film magnates and film stars.

Gershwin was attracted by beautiful women, and for him it was always difficult if not impossible to refuse the attentions of charming ladies. Although by no means a Don Juan, he went through many and various love affairs. He was, in fact, rather shy, almost prudish, and basically unsure of himself. He often fell deeply in love but, when the relationship had gone on for a while and the question of marriage began to crop up, he always found some excuse to escape it. The reason he gave for not marrying a famous singer, although he had seriously considered it, was that he had heard her play some of her own pieces on the piano. He knew he could not live with that sort of playing for the rest of his life! He rejected the idea of marrying one other eligible lady because he was doubtful of her morals, and he refused yet another because she came from a different class of society. One girl who was deeply in love with Gershwin decided to break with him for good because the most ardent declaration that he was able to give her was that she was good for his bad stomach.

Spastic Colitis, Chronic Neurosis, or Composer's Stomach?

Despite his strong physique, Gershwin was troubled for many years, before his fatal illness, by occasional attacks of nausea and vague stomach complaints that he could not precisely locate. From 1923 onward, he consulted one doctor after another for these symptoms. Gaining no relief, he consulted a psychiatrist and underwent psychoanalysis. None of this was of any use, and he continued to be plagued by the symptoms right up to his death.

Gershwin kept a careful journal of his diet, and he always hoped that he would himself be able to find out the cause of his diffuse stomach complaints. He tried out every conceivable diet and regimen, but all in vain—he never was able to cure his tormenting stomach complaints. Time and again he would complain, "I often have a nauseating feeling at the pit of my stomach and feel I'm going to be sick." Gershwin went on consulting doctors, but none of them succeeded in curing him. Various diagnoses were made of his condition, including spastic colitis, chronic neurosis, and composer's stomach.

An Emotional Change

Until 1936, Gershwin had always been an extrovert, loving the life that he led. As before, he was surrounded by friends, and he was still leading an active social life, just as during all the years before, when all at once he began to feel more and more isolated and lonely. Although previously he had avoided marriage by every possible means, now he was more and more often heard to say that he ought to get married. Once he sat down and wrote letters to old flames, inviting them to come see him in California. When none of them came, his feeling of loneliness grew even more pronounced.

At a large gala in 1936, Gershwin met Paulette Goddard, who was married to Charlie Chaplin, and he immediately fell in love with her. When he came home from this party, he felt convinced that this was the woman he wanted to marry. In the following weeks, he was entirely absorbed by a stormy love affair. When Paulette Goddard refused to leave Chaplin, it was a severe shock to Gershwin, intensifying his feeling of loneliness during the last few months of 1936.

The emotional change in him became more marked, and he began to grow irritable and touchy about matters to which previously he would not have attached the slightest importance.

Gershwin also began to worry about going bald, and he bought an appliance that was advertised as a cure for baldness (Fig 30). It consisted of a metal cap connected by a flexible tube to a motor-driven pump. The cap was placed over the scalp; the pump was then started to produce a suction effect on the scalp. Gershwin submitted to this vacuum treatment for at least half an hour a day, hoping thus to improve the growth of hair on his head.

Increasingly often, he began to sink into periods of melancholy, and one day in January 1937 he said to one of his closest friends, "I am 38 years old, wealthy and famous, but I'm still deeply unhappy. How come?" Outwardly, he was still a picture of health. His face was suntanned, his eyes were bright and lively, and his well-built, athletic body had lost none of its healthy appearance. Despite extensive and repeated medical examinations, his doctors could find nothing wrong with him. They considered that the symptoms were due to bad nerves and that they were only temporary. Not long afterward, however, further symptoms appeared of a nature suggesting that the patient was, in fact, seriously ill.

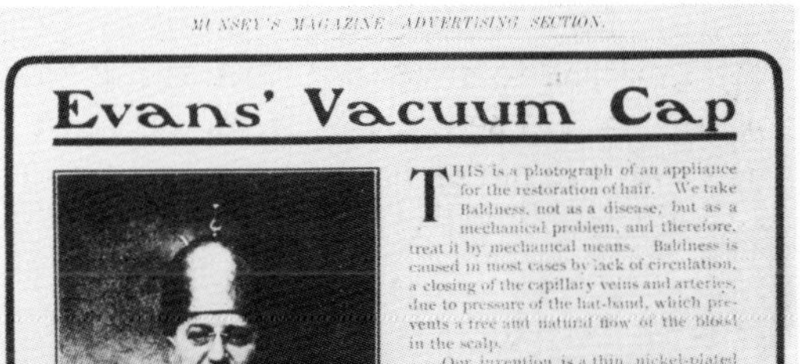

***Figure 30:** Evan's vacuum cap—an appliance for the restoration of hair. (From the* Munsey's Magazine *advertising section.)*

Uncinate Fits and Psychomotor Epilepsy

On February 11, 1937, Gershwin appeared with the Los Angeles Philharmonic Orchestra in a program entirely devoted to his works. While conducting his *Piano Concerto in F Major*, he suffered an attack, lasting only 10 or 20 seconds, during which he just passed out. There were no spasmodic jerks, and he remained upright, but he did miss several bars. As he returned to reality, he continued conducting just as if nothing had happened. Later, he said that, immediately preceding this momentary blackout, he had sensed a loathsome and repulsive smell as of burnt rubber, although this could not be traced to an irritation by any external stimulus.

In April 1937, Gershwin had a new epileptic manifestation. When he was sitting in a barber's chair in Beverly Hills, his consciousness became clouded and he more or less blacked out after experiencing the strange smell like burnt rubber. He estimated that this episode lasted something over half a minute. Gershwin mentioned these symptoms to his doctors, Gregory Zilboorg and his psychoanalyst colleague Dr. Ernest Simmel, who suggested that the cause of the symptoms was physical rather than psychogenic in origin.

Increased Intracranial Pressure

It was only in June 1937 that there were more obvious signs that Gershwin was seriously ill. A striking indifference and apathy came over him. And some mornings he would wake up in a dazed condition, appearing to be more or less muddleheaded. In the daytime, he would sometimes be troubled by a sensation that his surroundings were moving up and down. With increasing frequency, he was now heard to complain of a severe headache, most pronounced in the mornings. Gershwin was now working on his fourth motion picture, *The Goldwyn Follies*.

Once or twice, people found him sitting in his bed with a glazed stare, the curtains drawn against the light of day, which seemed to bother him. When asked, he could not say how long he had been sitting like that. He felt drained of all his energy and vitality, and the decision to get up from bed in the morning now called for an almost impossible effort.

His personal physician, who was also Greta Garbo's doctor, examined him time and again. As yet, Gershwin still had no discernible focal neurological deficits. None of Gershwin's closest friends understood how serious this headache was and misinterpreted the symptoms as being psychogenic. The symptoms were explained as "a neurotic protest against the artificial world of Hollywood" and so forth.

On June 12, Gershwin went on a holiday with a friend to Coronado. On arriving home again, he seemed to be virtually restored to his former self. For a short while, it looked as if those people who considered that Gershwin's symptoms were due to overwork and to an aversion to Hollywood would be proved right.

After a dinner given by Irving Berlin on Sunday, June 20, Gershwin, however, again complained of an intolerable headache. Two or three days later, he lunched with a group that included Paulette Goddard. His mental change was now more obvious. He seemed indifferent, apathetic, and somewhat slow-witted. For the keen observer, it would have been obvious that he showed a general bradyphrenia.

For the first time, his friends understood that he was seriously ill, and the next day they made arrangements to admit him to a hospital. There he underwent a neurological examination. The only demonstrable finding was hyposmia on the right side. There was no papilledema, and no visual field defect was discernible. The intention was to continue the examination with a lumbar puncture and an analysis of the cerebrospinal fluid, but this Gershwin refused, considering it to be far too painful.

The Final Phase

When Gershwin was discharged from the hospital, arrangements were made for a nurse to be with him all the time and he also received daily psychoanalytic treatment. Nonetheless, his condition worsened, becoming more and more alarming.

Late one evening, when George and Ira were returning home from a party given by Samuel Goldwyn, George sat down at the edge of the street with his feet in the gutter and put his head in his hands, complaining bitterly that his splitting headache and the repulsive smell of burnt rubber, which was now with him almost all of the time, were driving him crazy.

On a later occasion, the knife with which he was eating fell from his hand. At another meal, he lost control and was unable to bring his fork to his mouth, and he also spilled water out of his glass when trying to drink. Even at this point, no one seemed to have understood that Gershwin showed a progressive organic brain disease.

It was decided to isolate him completely in the hope that the full, undisturbed rest would cure his symptoms. He was given a room in a private nursing home in Beverly Hills under the continual supervision of his doctor and his own nurse. This complete rest apparently did him some good. He complained less of his headache, and now and again during the day he even sat down at the piano of his own accord, playing with evident enjoyment. When he tried, however, to play a piece for his doctor on July 8, he lost the coordination of his piano playing as well.

Brain Herniation, Diagnosis, and Operation

On July 9, Ira visited his brother, found him asleep, and decided to return later during the day. George did not wake up until five in the afternoon and was then so feeble that he had to call his nurse to help him out to the bathroom. On the way, he suddenly collapsed, losing consciousness immediately. He was at once taken to the hospital. On arrival, he was in a deep coma. He showed a left-sided hemiparesis, and there was also papilledema with severe protrusion.

Now, at last, everything was done to mobilize the foremost experts. Desperate attempts were made to reach Dr. Walter Dandy of The Johns Hopkins Hospital in Baltimore, at the time the most distinguished practicing neurosurgeon in the United States. But he was at sea, taking a holiday on a private yacht. A telegram was therefore sent to the White House, and two U.S. Navy destroyers put to sea; when the yacht had been located, Dr. Dandy was taken off in one of the destroyers and brought ashore. He was then taken with a special motorcycle escort to Cumberland and flown from there in a private plane to

Newark, there to take another private plane already waiting to fly him to Gershwin in Los Angeles. At the same time, contact had been established with another well-known neurosurgeon in California, Dr. Howard Nafziger. He, too, was on holiday, but was closer at hand at Lake Tahoe, from where he was immediately flown to Los Angeles.

Because it was not possible to establish the precise location of the suspected brain tumor, ventriculography was undertaken. This showed that both lateral ventricles were displaced far toward the left and, whereas the left lateral ventricle was basically normal in configuration, the right was greatly flattened and the right temporal horn was not filled at all. The intraventricular pressure had been very high. It was now obvious that there was a tumor in the right temporal region.

Dandy had by this time reached Newark, but there he was stopped by Nafziger. The latter conferred with Dandy over the telephone and informed him that an immediate operation was imperative and that by the time Dandy arrived, the operation would be over.

Late on the evening of July 10, immediately after the ventriculography, Gershwin was taken to the operating room. Nafziger and Carl Rand explored a partially cystic glioma in the temporal lobe and performed a partial resection. Microscopic examination revealed a "spongioblastoma multiforme" (that is, with today's nomenclature, a malignant glioma). The operation was concluded just after midnight. Without regaining consciousness after the brain herniation, Gershwin died on the morning of July 11, 1937.

Announcing his death on the radio, the commentator stated, "The man who said he had more notes in his head than he could write down in a hundred years died suddenly today in Hollywood."

Epicrisis

Not infrequently, the initial symptoms of a temporal lobe tumor are attacks of psychomotor epilepsy, which are easily misinterpreted as psychogenic symptoms. In the case of a more slowly infiltrating astrocytoma in the temporal lobe, brief sporadic attacks of the type that plagued Gershwin, initiated by uncinate fits, may for a long time be the sole symptom. The patient may easily be given the wrong diagnosis (for example, psychoneurosis or hysteria), and his symptoms may cause him to become severely paranoid.

What is interesting in Gershwin's case history is the occurrence, over many years, of sporadic attacks of nausea and unpleasant sensations in the pit of the stomach. Gershwin consulted many doctors about this problem, and they gave every conceivable diagnosis, including chronic neurosis, spastic colitis, and composer's stomach. One common symptom in temporal lobe epilepsy is a visceral aura or "rising epigastric sensation" from the pit of the stomach, accompanied by nausea and followed by a brief clouding of consciousness. If such a rising epigastric sensation recurs as an aura always accompanying an attack of clouded consciousness, this is a strong indication that the cause is located in the temporal lobe.

One may speculate that, in the case of Gershwin, there was initially a low grade astrocytoma in the right temporal lobe that caused abortive temporal lobe seizures with a rising epigastric sensation. Then, in the final phase, this astrocytoma may have undergone rapid malignant degeneration and turned into a fulminating glioblastoma multiform.

Gershwin passed away when he was at the height of his career. Only near the end did it become clear to his physicians that he had a brain tumor. By the time of this diagnosis, there was with all certainty already irreversible cerebral damage secondary to the brain herniation.

This was in the year 1937—and at the age of only 38, Gershwin was one of the most successful composers that the United States had ever produced. He had made a fortune on his music, and his pieces were being sung, whistled, and played by millions upon millions of people in the United States and Europe. Even so, his admirers could scarcely have imagined how his popularity was to rise to even greater heights in years to come. Eight years after his death, *Rhapsody in Blue* (1924) was played in Moscow, and the following year it was performed in Prague by Eugene List and the Czechoslovak Philharmonic Orchestra conducted by Leonard Bernstein.

Gershwin wrote the first great American opera, *Porgy and Bess.* His too are the melodies *Swanee, I Got Rhythm, Somebody Loves Me, Oh, Lady Be Good, Embraceable You, Fascinating Rhythm, It Ain't Necessarily So, Love Is Here to Stay, The Man I Love, They Can't Take That Away from Me,* and many more.

Unfortunately, the pathogenesis of cerebral gliomas remains veiled in obscurity. It is obvious that these tumors develop long before they give rise to clinical manifestations of their existence. We still do not know how long they have been present before they are detected. The prognosis for these terrible growths is as gloomy now as in Gershwin's day. The only progress has been in improved diagnostic methods.

Had Gershwin had his tumor today, he would most probably have had to suffer less because his brain tumor would certainly have been diagnosed much earlier than was the case half a century ago. Nonetheless, the final outcome would have been the same.

As Dandy explained his view to the doctors in charge of the case, "It was just one of those fulminating tumors. Although the tumor might have been extirpated and he would have recovered for a little while, it would have recurred very quickly. I think the outcome is much the best for himself. For a man as brilliant as he with a recurring tumor, life would have been terrible; it would have been a slow death."

Selected References

1. Armitage M. *George Gershwin: Man and Legend.* New York, NY: Duell, Sloan and Pearce, Van Rees Press; 1958.

2. Carp L. George Gershwin—illustrious American composer: His fatal glioblastoma. *Am J Surg Pathol.* 1979;3:473-478.

3. Duke V. *Passport to Paris.* Boston, Mass: Little, Brown and Co; 1955.

4. Ewen D. *A Journey to Greatness: The Life and Music of George Gershwin.* New York, NY: Henry Holt and Co; 1956.

5. Fabricant ND. George Gershwin's fatal headache. *Eye Ear Nose Throat Mon.* 1958;37:332-334.

6. Fabricant ND. *Thirteen Famous Patients.* Philadelphia, Pa: Chilton Book Co; 1960.

7. Gardner LD. George Gershwin. *Br Med J.* 1979;2:1368.

8. Goldberg I. *George Gershwin.* New York, NY: Simon and Schuster Inc; 1931.

9. Ljunggren B. The case of George Gershwin. *Neurosurgery*. 1982;10:733-736.

10. Matthew-Walker R. *Rachmaninoff*. London, England; 1984:6-7.

11. Minerva news and notes. Views. *Br Med J*. 1979;2:1007.

12. Schwartz C. *Gershwin: His Life & Music*. New York, NY: Da Capo; 1973.

13. Trethowan WH. Music and mental disorder. In: Critchley M, Henson RA, eds. *Music and the Brain*. London, England: William Heinemann Medical Books Limited; 1977:342.

Chapter 8

The Case of the Sleepy Sea Lord

On June 27, 1942, a huge Anglo-American convoy of merchant ships laden below their marks with tanks, aircraft, ammunition, food, and other war necessities, left Iceland. Their destination was Archangel in northern Russia. At this time, Stalin's armies were fighting a desperate battle against Hitler's armies, which were advancing and winning on all fronts.

When clear, the appointed heavy naval escort met these merchant ships north of Iceland and formed up to establish their own screening positions. The 17th Russian-bound convoy—covering roughly the area of Hyde Park in London—was on its way.

On July 4, when the convoy was in enemy waters protected by German U-boats and torpedo-bombers based in northern Norway, the escort commanders were ordered to withdraw at high speed and the convoy captains to scatter the convoy by some murderous radio signals transmitted from some 2,000 miles away. This resulted in a terrible disaster. Twenty-three of the merchant ships and their cargoes still lie sprawled and wrecked in the waters of the Arctic Circle on the Barents seabed. Only 11 of the ships reached their destination. Winston Churchill called convoy PQ 17 "one of the most melancholy naval episodes in the whole war." Stalin wondered if the British navy had lost all sense of glory.

These murderous signals were sent against all advice by the first sea lord of the British Admiralty, Sir Dudley Pound, who at the time had already exhibited severe symptoms of mental exhaustion and also possibly brain destruction. Had Pound not been held in such high esteem by Churchill, possibly other admirals would have forced him to consult a physician at an earlier stage. Pound died on Trafalgar Day, in 1943, from a glioma, possibly originating in the basal ganglia of the left cerebral hemisphere.

Background

History records many instances of mentally unfit men making important decisions with serious consequences for millions of people. When Churchill replaced Neville Chamberlain in May 1940, Chamberlain's physical and mental buoyancy was already failing. Two months later, he underwent a surgical exploration, which revealed an inoperable rectal cancer. He died in November 1940, persuaded that German troups would land in England.

The British ambassador in Washington, Lord Lothian, showed even more prominent symptoms and signs of failing cognition. Apart from the habit of falling asleep on duty, once at a banquet, he surprised American journalists upon his arrival in the United States in November 1940 by declaring, "Well boys, Britain's broke; it's your money we want." He had chronic uremia and died within two weeks.

At the British Admiralty, Sir Roger Backhouse was the first sea lord immediately preceding the outbreak of World War II. Toward the end of 1938, those around him were shocked when Backhouse's personality suddenly changed; at times he would speak in a vulgar and objectionable way. He would refer to his long-serving secretary as "that lazy, young bitch," behavior far removed from his previous well-bred and polite manner. During the early months of 1939, he did little work and gradually seemed more powerless, absentminded, and apathetic.

After a period of convalescence at sea, he appeared to be his former self (compare George Gershwin, see Chapter 7), but soon relapsed after his return to the Admiralty. Toward the end of April 1939, a severe mental disturbance was obvious. He had become increasingly inattentive, confused, and even lethargic. Lord Stanhope, then first lord of the Admiralty, lacked any real knowledge of the sea, ships, and naval strategy, but he should be given credit for arranging a medical examination of the sick admiral. It was obvious to the distinguished neurologist Dr. (later Sir) Frances Walshe that Backhouse had a rapidly growing brain tumor. The diagnosis of a frontal malignant glioma was established and the commander-in-chief of the British Mediterranean Fleet, Admiral Sir Dudley Pound, was summoned home to fill the vital gap. Soon afterward, Backhouse died without even knowing that he had been replaced.

Admiral Dudley Pound and Winston Churchill

Pound had begun his naval career in January 1891 when he was 13 years old. He had been fond of horses as a boy and wanted to join the cavalry, but one day, while standing on Stokes Bay pier in Spithead, a naval cutter came in under sail and glided alongside the pier. Young Dudley was impressed, transferred his allegiance from horses to ships, and duly joined the Royal Navy as a cadet.

In the naval college, and later in the Victorian Fleet with its traditions and strict discipline, he received his first training. There he learned to obey and, on request, to rattle off the long list of faults that would result in corporal punishment for the young cadets, or "snotties," who were left in no doubt that they represented the lowest form of life at sea.

On his 19th birthday, Pound was promoted to sublieutenant, and after steady progress he was made captain in command of HMS Colossus at the Battle of Jutland in May 1916, the 17th in Admiral Jellicoe's long, oblique file of 24 capital ships. Some shells certainly struck Colossus and one man lost his arm, but the damage inflicted was indeed minor when compared with the total losses. Colossus scored several hits on enemy vessels and her captain was mentioned in dispatches.

Pound's signal officer at Jutland recalled half a century later that life on Colossus had always seemed dull, though Pound was agreeable, courteous, and friendly. He seemed completely preoccupied by higher things and his task of making Colossus the finest ship in the fleet. One of the "snotties" on board Colossus was Jack Broome, who 26 years later was to play a tragic role in a disaster that was caused by Pound. Broome has no recollection of Pound but remembers that he liked his bulldog and that service on Colossus was similar to being a miner in a collier's holdblack, cold, exhausting, and "getting six on the backside" every night for a week for lighting a cigarette without asking the sublieutenant's permission.

During the interwar years, Pound climbed farther up the career ladder. He committed no blunders but, on the other hand, he showed no unusual brilliance. He was a tremendous worker, had no hobbies except hunting and fishing, and was unable to relax into any sort of humorous pose. He has been described as remarkably narrow-minded, without a thought beyond naval affairs, and soon out of his element if the conversation strayed from service topics. Although a dedicated man, he had a limited horizon, which did not include a knowledge of human relations, international politics, or the effects of his words and deeds upon others. There was a conspicuous absence of books in Pound's cabin.

He had just been installed as first sea lord when World War II broke out and Lord Stanhope was replaced by Churchill. When the newly appointed first lord and first sea lord met on the day war broke out, the omens for good collaboration and a harmonious relationship were not particularly favorable. The British Mediterranean Fleet had been dispersed to various ports when Mussolini seized Albania on Good Friday of 1939. Pound's failure to concentrate the fleet provoked Churchill to caustic criticism in the House of Commons; Churchill did not accept a failure in Whitehall intelligence as the explanation. However, against the odds, the combination of Churchill* and the conscientious first sea lord turned out to be most successful.

Soon Churchill formed a close attachment to, and trust in, Pound, who was cold, remote, and without much humor, though he was basically a humble man with none of the arrogance that marked many of the earlier 20th century British admirals. Pound quickly developed an intense loyalty toward Churchill, was never heard to criticize him or to complain about him, and would not tolerate opposition to the continuous stream of ideas, reproofs, "prayers," and "proddings" that emanated from the first lord's room. Churchill's demand of total and uncritical acceptance by his colleagues and associates was a posture from which Pound rarely diverged.

From Pound's experience of war, limited to service as captain of Colossus at Jutland, two characteristics evolved: emphasis on the importance of guns and the capital ship, and direct interference by the Admiralty with operational commanders. The first sea lord, "a supreme centralizer, wedded to the battle fleet concept," turned out to be prone to backseat driving, sometimes with disastrous results. He could never fully realize that times had changed so that both guns and battleships were on the way out and that the burden of naval war would fall upon smaller ships, carriers, and submarines.

The so-called "phony war" annoyed Churchill, but at sea the war was real from the first day. After only a month, the partnership between Churchill and Pound had to endure its first ordeal. It was after that nightmare when Kapitän zur See Günther Prien boldly succeeded in slipping his U-boat (U-47) through the Kirk Sound into Scapa Flow in the Orkneys. Undiscovered, U-47 fired her torpedoes and sank HMS Royal Oak, and 833 officers and men of the Royal Navy and Royal Marines met their death in a harbor where they believed themselves safe.

The next morning, Pound had to face Churchill and explain his failure at not having made Prien's task impossible. Rear Admiral Servaes remembered the occasion "only too well. I was with Sir Dudley Pound when Churchill came into the room to be given details of the disaster. Instead of recriminations as to why the base was not better defended, all he said was 'What a wonderful feat of arms.'"

Beginning in October 1939, the Royal Navy began to scour the Atlantic for the devastating surface raider, the heavily armored German "pocket battleship" Graf Spee. Churchill took a keen interest in the operation. After having been damaged by three British cruisers in action off the River Plate, Graf Spee sought refuge in Montevideo and four days later was scuttled outside the harbor. Churchill was in ecstatic spirits during those days and hardly left the map room, which was the center of activity.

Then, when victory was won, Churchill hastened to exploit the success of the first sea lord and his associates. In a delighted broadcast to the nation, Churchill depicted the

*To his last days, Pound maintained his great respect for Churchill, to the point of addressing him as "sir," instead of the traditional "first lord," or after May 10, 1940, "prime minister."

thrilling pursuit of Graf Spee and how eventually she was surrounded and doomed. As he was managing to inspire the nation with this speech, the broadcast also became a foundation stone for his career as one of the world's most powerful politicians and military leaders.

Captured British crews, who had been kept on Graf Spee, had been transferred to a German tanker, Altmark, which at first hid in the South Atlantic. In mid-February 1940, she sought refuge in a fiord on the south coast of neutral Norway, where two British destroyers kept watch on her. Without informing the admiral in command of operations in this area, Churchill made the British Admiralty order the boarding of Altmark to release the prisoners. This was a flagrant breach of neutrality and most certainly dictated by political motives.

The successful mission received great publicity and undoubtedly strenghtened Churchill's position. That the operation was performed with Pound's nodded assent shows how the two men thought and acted alike. It does not indicate any great indulgence from Pound. He behaved at the Admiralty as he had done on sea, according to the maxim that the captain knows best and consequently commands without having to consult or inform anyone else, and certainly not a subordinate.

Pound was rather deaf, and Churchill may have found this useful, because Pound did not like to admit that he had not heard what Churchill said and would nod his head to statements with which he might have otherwise disagreed. Liddel Hart noted in December 1939 that Chatfield (minister for the Coordination of Defense) suffered from deafness so that he was apt to miss the point in discussion, while Pound was even deafer as well as stupid.

On one occasion, General Ironside (chief of the Imperial General Staff) tackled Winston about the soldiers who had been lost in the sinking of the SS Yorkshire. Winston referred the question to Pound, who started looking through his papers and gave a series of irrelevant figures—it emerged that they were the quantities of oil stored at various places—he having apparently only caught the word "Yorkshire" and not the subject of the discussion.

However, against such unfavorable and deprecatory judgments, stand testimonies that Pound showed unshakable calm and unlimited patience. He never seemed pressed for time or cut short other officers, even if their reports were of secondary importance. His questions were shrewd and very much to-the-point. Pound always had to grasp every detail of the subject under discussion.

It seems justifiable to conclude that Pound was not subservient to Churchill and that he really accomplished a good deal simply by praiseworthy handling of his defiant colleague. One of Churchill's many brainstorms was a plan to send a fleet of surface ships into the Baltic to cut off the supplies of Swedish ore to Germany and secure the Baltic. He was fond of imaginative code names for his wild plans, and this one, which according to senior naval officers was crazy and could only have ended in catastrophe, he called "Operation Catherine" after the Russian empress, Catherine the Great.

To Churchill "Operation Catherine" was "the supreme naval offensive open to the Royal Navy." In fact, this plan, which he presented to the Admiralty on the third day after the outbreak of World War II, had been maturing in his brain for at least 25 years. In the summer of 1914, Churchill had proposed that the War Office investigate the possibility of the British Fleet moving into the Baltic to secure naval bases. The 1939 operation had every earmark of becoming a repeat of Lord Fisher's and Churchill's costly failure at the Dardanelles a quarter of a century earlier.

Fortunately, Pound handled Churchill's obsession, not by completely rejecting it, but by allowing the planning to continue while he sent repeated memoranda to Churchill expressing serious objections. At the beginning of 1940, Pound sent a paper to Churchill intended "to make his flesh creep," depicting all the hazards and ending with a "most strongly" presented conclusion that all special preparations should be discontinued. Churchill fought back and it was not until the German invasion of Denmark and Norway that the "brainstorm" was finally discarded.

At the end of 1939, Churchill suggested that a British expeditionary force should occupy the ore fields in the Gällivare area in northern Sweden. In a Christmas Day minute to Pound, Churchill asked what the navy's contribution could be. Pound's reply must have discomforted Churchill: Pound answered that any such attack must be written off if the war at sea were not to be lost "with the reduced forces we should have outside the Baltic."

Pound's Failing Health

It is difficult, if not impossible, to pinpoint when Pound began to exhibit symptoms of the cerebral glioma that he would die from in October 1943. As early as the spring of 1940, it was obvious that he was somnolent. A staff officer remembered a meeting when he sat near Pound, "After a not very long time, I noticed that Pound was drooling down the stem of his pipe—not just a drop, for I was at least five yards away. He may not have been asleep but he was quite out for the count."

The director of naval intelligence became seriously concerned about Pound's health. He would see him three or four times a week, and regularly every Tuesday morning when the directors of intelligence of all three services met with the chiefs of staff.

That Pound used to doze was common knowledge, but the director of naval intelligence said, "What I find hard to believe is that he was mentally awake the whole time and was automatically alerted with full knowledge of what had been said and was taking place, by the mention of anything to do with the Fleet. In any case, this seems to me irrelevant as the three chiefs of staff met in order to bring their collective wisdom, experience, and views to bear on all questions and not only those concerning their own service. They were discreet and tactful and were just as conscious as I of Pound's infirmity. Although it had not occurred to them that he was already a sick man, they were alive to the fact that his memory, judgment, and mental alertness, but not the power of decision, were waning. But neither was prepared to undertake the thankless task I had in mind for them."

Pound's former flag captain from Colossus had been in the furniture trade in the interwar period but had been called up and appointed duty signal officer. Pound would sometimes visit the lower war room next door to the small operations room in the basement where four officers, including his former flag captain, were on watch.

The former flag captain was somewhat surprised when Pound once told him that he could not understand why he had not reached a higher command. He was later to state that Pound "seemed vague about the passage of time in that I had had 18 years in commerce and it was over 20 years since we had met."

In the summer of 1940, Britain feared a German invasion. The attention of British intelligence was concentrated on preparations for this plan, "Operation Seelöwe." It was not until the end of October that the director of naval intelligence received completely reliable information that the German invasion was off, except as a diversionary threat. Pound was then immediately notified.

In March 1941, Pound was informed that Britain could no longer count on this state of immunity. It was then that the chief of naval intelligence was greatly surprised when Pound answered that he had never been told that the threat of invasion had receded during the previous October. Pound's vagueness about the passage of time and forgetfulness in a matter of supreme importance are indications of an early destructive lesion in his brain.

Sir Arthur Bryant, quoting from Field Marshal Lord Alanbrooke's diary, remarked how by the autumn of 1941 "the First Sea Lord was growing old and tired," and that Alanbrooke found the chiefs of staff (COS) committee got through its business far more quickly "in the chairman's (i.e. Pound's) absence." He then quoted further evidence from the diary, dated February 17, 1942, "Am getting more and more worried by old Dudley Pound as First Sea Lord. With him it is impossible for the COS to perform the functions it should in the biggest Imperial War we are ever likely to be engaged in. He is asleep 75 percent of the time he should be working."

"A futile meandering COS meeting," the diary notation for February 18 begins, "with practically no major points and with Dudley Pound half asleep." Pound used to spend his nights on a campbed at the Admiralty and, when he dosed off in committee, "he looked like an old parrot asleep on his perch," Alanbrooke observed.

Sir Stafford Cripps, the leader of the House of Commons, had long been dissatisfied with the direction the war was taking, and in September 1942, he felt such discord with Churchill that he could no longer delay his resignation. In the correspondence which followed, the prime minister challenged him to name those in whom he had no confidence. Cripps bluntly replied that Pound was beyond his ability to work. Churchill was pained by this attack on Pound to whom he had long been deeply attached (Fig 31).

At the Casablanca Conference, Churchill and Roosevelt and their chiefs of staff met to discuss the planned invasion of southern Italy. On January 21, 1943, Alanbrooke noted in his diary that, "We had had many debates on the relative advantages of Sardinia and Sicily . . . and it was only at the end of much hard work that I obtained general agreement of Sicily. And now suddenly the joint planning staff reappeared on the scene with a strong preference for Sardinia and expressing most serious doubts as to our ability on the Sicilian operation. They had carried with them Mountbatten (Vice-Admiral Lord Louis Mountbatten); 'Peter' Portal (the then Air Marshal Sir Charles Portal, chief of air staff) and 'Pug' Ismay (Churchill's personal staff officer and head of the War Cabinet secretariat) were beginning to waver, and dear old Dudley Pound was, as usual, asleep and with no views either way."

And from the Casablanca Conference General George S. Patton made a similar notation in his war diary dated January 16: "Sir Dudley Pound, Field Marshal Alanbrooke, and General Marshall and his wife came to dinner. I walked home with the Marshalls. Pound slept most of the dinner. The more I see of the so-called Great, the less they impress me. I am better."

No measures seem to have been undertaken to replace the first sea lord, despite his crucial position and obvious unfitness. However, early in the summer of 1943, Pound became aware that something was wrong with the function of his right foot and hand. He discreetly sent for a physician (the consultant neurologist to the Royal Navy) who found a definite right-sided hemiparesis, and since Pound's condition seemed so alarming, he

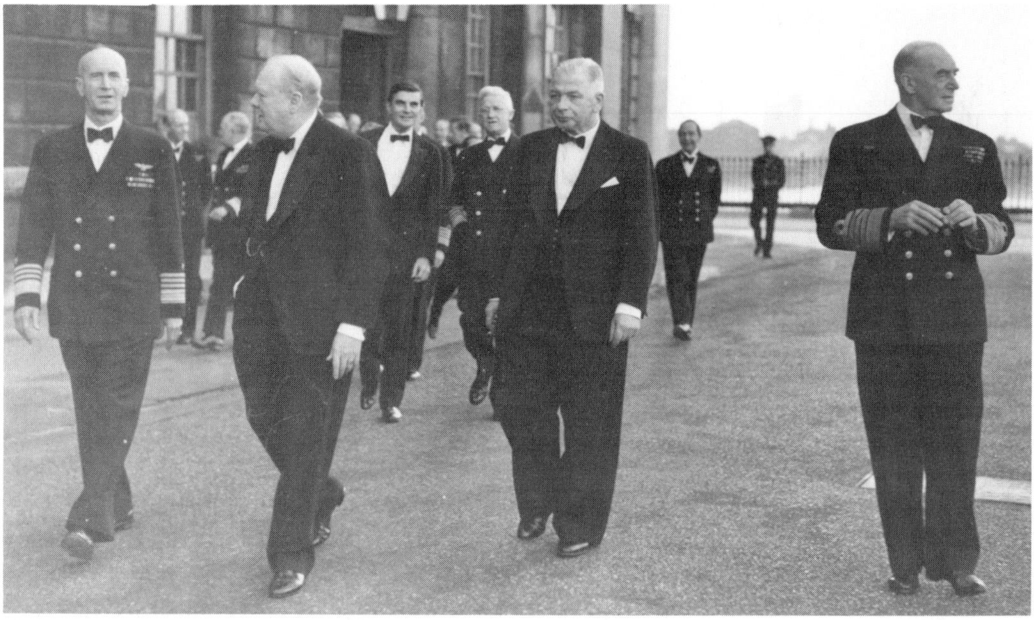

Figure 31: *Prime Minister Winston Churchill with his successor as first lord of the Admiralty, A. V. Alexander, to his left. To his further left is the first sea lord, Sir Dudley Pound. To the right, U.S. Admiral Ernest King, chief of American naval operations. Taken at the Royal Naval College, Greenwich, September, 1942. (Prime Minister Churchill had invited himself to this dinner meeting, which was intended to be a strictly naval occasion!)*

sent a strongly worded personal letter to the medical director-general stating that Pound was unfit and refused to listen to medical advice.

Pound was aggressive, unappreciative, and unreasonable and would not accept the advice to cancel his plans to attend the Quebec Conference with Churchill. However, no action was taken and the physician's letter was not even acknowledged by the medical director-general.

In August 1943, Churchill and Pound, and their entourage, including Sir Charles Wilson (later Lord Moran), Churchill's personal physician, left Britain on board the Queen Mary bound for Halifax, Nova Scotia. During a sight-seeing trip before the Quebec Conference, Mountbatten literally saved Pound's life when Pound lost his balance on the edge of a ravine; there was great difficulty in getting him back to the car.

Churchill later stated that he had been somewhat astonished by Pound's poor appearance at the Quebec Conference (Fig 32): "I had noticed that Admiral Pound had not gone with the other two chiefs of staff to the lake, and I suggested that he should come with us now. His staff officer said that he had a lot of cleaning up to do after the conference. I had been surprised by the subdued part he had taken in the far-running naval discussions, but when he said that he could not come fishing I had a fear that all was not well."

After the Quebec Conference, Churchill went to Washington to see President Roosevelt. In his diary for September 9, Moran notes that "stories have been going that Dudley Pound drops off to sleep in important committees, even at meetings with the Cabinet. . . . It does not seem much of a compliment to this sailor if they can detect no difference be-

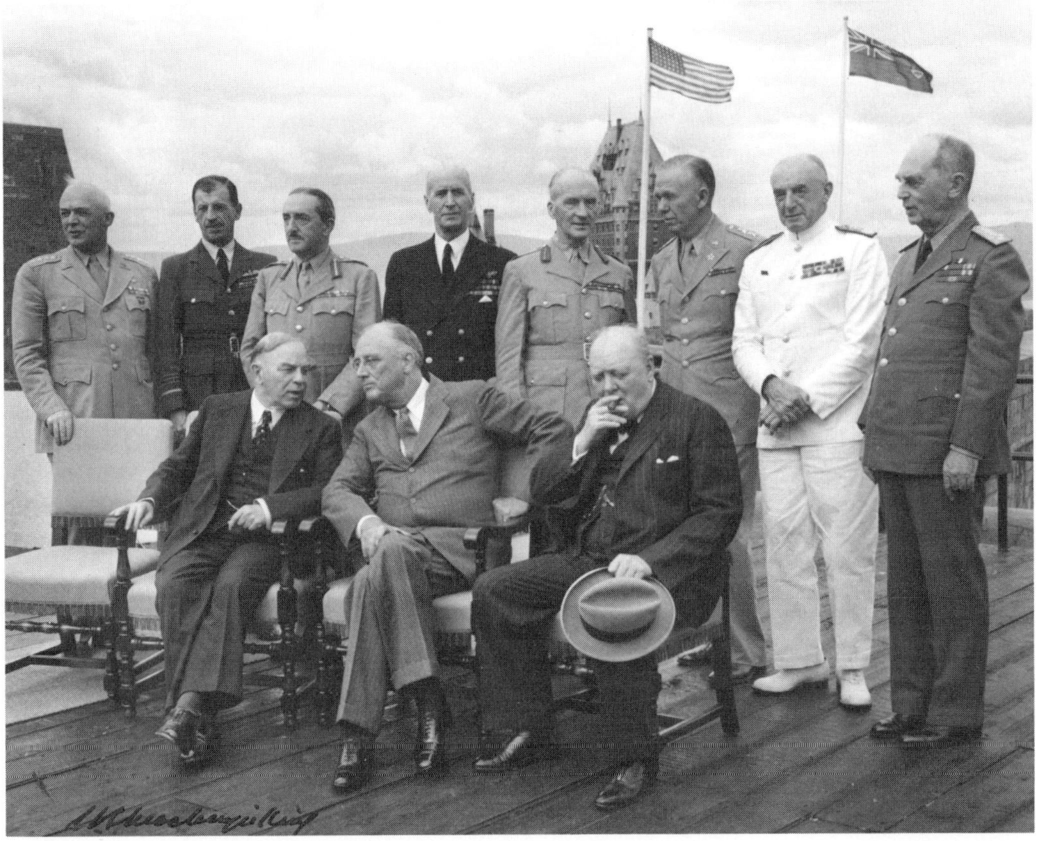

Figure 32: *The Anglo-American "top brass" at the Quebec Conference in early September, 1943. In the front, W. L. Mackenzie King, prime minister of Canada, President Roosevelt, and Winston Churchill. The admiral in the white uniform is Sir Dudley Pound and the general behind Mackenzie King (third man from left) is Field Marshal Viscount Alanbrooke.*

tween his mental process now, when he is a very sick man, and the time when he was fit and well. . . . I first noticed this at the Guildhall one morning during a freedom ceremony when I happened to be seated on the platform next to Pound, and noticed that he had fallen asleep; his head had sunk until it almost touched my shoulder. As for the prime minister, he does not notice this kind of thing until it hits him. And here at Washington it has hit him pretty hard."

That same day, Churchill sent for Moran and declared that he was worried about Pound who, on the previous night after dinner, had come to see him and President Roosevelt. Roosevelt had asked him some very ordinary questions and Churchill was surprised that Pound's answers were "wide of the mark." Churchill then asked Pound if he really meant what he had just said whereupon Pound sat up straight and stated that he would let Churchill have a full report in the morning. He then rose, said that he felt tired, and would go to bed. Churchill told Moran that Roosevelt had remarked that at some of the meetings Pound appeared torpid and he had decided that Pound was finished.

The next morning, Pound came to see Churchill. At that meeting Pound abruptly told Churchill that he had come to resign because he no longer felt able to carry out his duties and had to be relieved; Pound explained that his right foot did not work properly and his hand was affected so that he could not even write his own name. According to Churchill's postwar memoirs, Pound concluded by saying, "I thought it would pass off, but it gets worse every day and I am no longer fit for duty."

Pound's Last Days

On the homeward voyage in the battleship Renown, Churchill "saw little of Sir Dudley Pound, except for a few chats on deck, as he kept to his cabin." It so happened that the first man on board upon arrival in Britain to welcome Churchill and his mission was Pound's former signal officer from the Jutland days, David Joel. He helped Pound into the boat to take him ashore and stayed with him in the drawing room car of the VIP train waiting for the prime minister and his party.

Joel commented, "It seemed that Pound's brain had gone and he was wandering. Though his mind had broken on current affairs he seemed perfectly lucid in speaking of the old Grand Fleet days. Somehow he took it for granted that I was with him. The intervening years were forgotten.

Pound spent his last days at the Royal Masonic Hospital in London. He underwent a minute clinical examination by the distinguished British neurologist, Sir Charles Symonds, who formed the opinion that the patient suffered from a glioma in the left cerebral hemisphere. Apart from the long history of increased somnolence and decrease in mental alertness, the patient showed a progressive right-sided hemiparesis and expressive dysphasia, together with bilateral papilloedema. Later, Sir Hugh Cairns also saw the patient and totally agreed with Symond's opinion. Both found the diagnosis of an inoperable mass sufficiently clear to obviate further investigation and felt "that air studies or angiography might cause aggravation of the dysphasia, which was Sir Dudley's most troublesome symptom."

Churchill saw Pound the day before he died. "His face was set," the prime minister told Lord Moran, imitating Pound's expressionless countenance: "He could not speak. But he took my hand, and when I said things that might be agreeable to him, he gripped it hard. His mind was all right; he knew what I was saying. He died on Trafalgar Day." Churchill meditated, then concluded, "Death is the greatest gift God has made to us."

Further Considerations

Terrible mistakes would almost certainly have been avoided had only Pound been forced to resign or at least to consult a physician early in 1941. A close description of two naval disasters, both of which had elements of a Greek tragedy, seems relevant, focusing on the role played by Pound.

The Life and Death of the Bismarck

The pursuit and sinking of the heavily armored German battleship, Bismarck, a massive floating gun platform with a displacement exceeding 50,000 metric tons and a crew of 103 officers and 1,962 petty officers and men, took place in May 1941, and was enacted over an immense area of ocean, from the Baltic to the Arctic, the Arctic to the Atlantic, and the Atlantic to the Bay of Biscay.

The chief of staff to the head of the Swedish Secret Service in Stockholm was an anti-Nazi. Through his contacts with the Norwegian military attaché in Stockholm, the British naval attaché there was able to warn the Admiralty in London on May 20 that the Swedish carrier Gotland had sighted six hours earlier two large German warships in the Kattegat on a northwest course. Pound's suspicion that these German heavy ships were preparing to break out into the Atlantic was confirmed the next day by air reconnaissance photography over a Norwegian fiord where the Bismarck was trying to hide.

The Admiralty in London was connected with Admiral Tovey, commander-in-chief of the British Home Fleet, by a direct telephone link to his flagship, King George V, moored at Scapa Flow. Once informed, Tovey immediately brought his fleet to readiness.

The first clash came early in the morning of May 24 when the Bismarck had just managed to dash through the Denmark Strait into the Atlantic. There she met the pride of the Royal Navy, the British battle cruiser Hood, the fastest warship of her size and once the largest in the world. In her first engagement, and after firing for only six minutes, the Bismarck blew the famous warship into two pieces "like a huge Chinese Christmas cracker." The Hood's destruction was certainly influenced by the fact that she carried a number of cordite-filled rockets that had made the stowage of ammunition difficult and dangerous. These rockets, which were untried new antiaircraft devices, had been another obsession of Churchill's; after the Hood tragedy, no further Churchill contraptions were installed into ships and the few already fitted were removed.

After the Bismarck's victory, the Royal Navy desperately sought to avenge the loss in a dramatic pursuit, deploying no less than 42 warships, including four battleships and two battle cruisers. The eventual "twilight of the gods" for the dreaded battleship and most of her crew cannot be ascribed, however, to a master brain in control of the gigantic operation. On the contrary, one may conclude that the victory was won despite the interference of the Admiralty and Pound, who sent several extraordinary messages to both Tovey and other admirals involved in the operation.

Pound's role in the drama showed no tactical genius but was characterized by inflexibility and clumsiness. His signals ranged from obvious pointers to stupid questions. He sent instructions to Tovey that he wanted some of his officers court-martialed for failing to engage Bismarck in battle when, in fact, this was exactly what the commander-in-chief of the Home Fleet had intended, so that he could bide for a better opportunity to attack. Tovey was so annoyed by Pound's insinuations of a lack of offensive spirit in his admirals that he signaled to the Admiralty that if necessary he would haul down his flag.

In another signal, Tovey was informed by Pound that the Bismarck must be sunk at whatever cost and that, if necessary, he, Tovey, must stay on the scene, even if it meant towing his flagship. This was a remarkable signal, drafted by Pound's strong-willed chief at 10 Downing Street, Churchill, who had become completely obsessed with sinking the Bismarck. Nevertheless, it had been approved by Pound.

The Arctic Convoys

On the same day that the Wehrmacht invaded the Soviet Union, Churchill in a broadcast promised all possible help from Britain. Two weeks later, he repeated his offer in a personal message to Stalin. Through his ambassador in London, Ivan Maisky, Stalin in early September 1941 urged Churchill to relieve the pressure exerted by the Nazi armies on the Soviet Union by creating a second front either in the Balkan States or in France, and by immediately sending 30,000 tons of aluminium for aircraft construction and at least 400 aircraft and 500 tanks every month beginning in October.

Later that same month, Churchill and Roosevelt sent their emissaries, Lord Beaverbrook and Averell Harriman, both with impeccable capitalist credentials, to negotiate with the Communist dictator, and on October 1 the treaty was signed. Beaverbrook read the long list of war materials, ranging from small warships, aircraft, trucks, jeeps, tanks, and medical equipment to 400,000 pairs of military boots monthly, which the United States and Britain pledged to send promptly. He then asked Stalin if he was content. "I am delighted," Stalin replied, while the reserved Russian minister, Maksim Litvinov, enthusiastically declared that now the war against Hitler's Reich could surely be won.

Stalin wanted the supplies to be delivered through Murmansk and Archangel in northern Russia and was not in favor of the far easier and more efficient route via the Persian Gulf because he did not wish any extension of British and American influence in that region. He declared that the Persian route was not advisable due to bad road and railway conditions, a statement which Churchill and Roosevelt accepted.

The arctic route was an extremely unsound route from a naval point of view, and the chances for survival of the crews of any sunken ships were small. The climatic conditions were appalling, with ferocious gales, ice, and fog, besides perpetual darkness for half the year and, in summer, perpetual day when there could be no respite from enemy attack. The wartime voyage took from 10 to 14 days, during most of which time the ships were within easy reach of German air and submarine bases in northern Norway. However, less than 8 percent of the 780 ships that completed the voyage to northern Russia in 42 convoys between August 1941 and May 1945 were sunk.

At the British Admiralty, Commander P. Q. Roberts organized the arctic convoys and, since he was known as "PQ," the outgoing convoys got this prefix while the homeward bound convoys were designated "QP," the reverse combination of his initials.

By the spring of 1942, the 12th convoy, PQ 12, had sailed and only one ship out of the 103 that had made the passage to northern Russia had been sunk. But with spring and better weather, the enemy gained an increasing advantage. The ice barrier had not receded far enough north for the convoys to give northern Norway, with its German submarine and air bases, a wide berth.

Tovey, one of whose chief commitments was to ensure the safe passage of the convoys, pointed out to Pound that they might well reach a scale beyond the escorting resources of the Home Fleet, and early in May 1942 Pound warned the cabinet's defense committee that conditions in the Arctic were moving so much in the enemy's favor that a temporary halt would seem the best solution.

Political pressure for their continuation, however, was exerted on Churchill by both Washington and Moscow. Roosevelt informed Churchill that the United States had made a "tremendous effort" and, at the end of April, had 107 ships fully loaded and ready to sail for Russia. At the same time, Stalin demanded that Churchill "take all possible measures" to ensure that the supplies reach the Soviet Union without delay. Churchill felt obliged to keep the promise he had made, and despite the great risk, he gave his personal directive that convoy PQ 17 should set sail in June.

The Curtain is Hoisted for Another Naval Drama

The intended departure date was June 11, but the need to relieve Malta had made such demands on the strength of the Home Fleet that the Archangel convoy was postponed for 16 days. The convoy consisted of 34 merchant ships; two-thirds were American, carrying 157,000 tons of tanks, aircraft, ammunition, food, and other war materials. On the afternoon of June 27, the convoy slipped out of Hvalfiord in Iceland in single file "and like as many dirty ducks, they waddled out past the nets and out to sea."

Not only did the size of the convoy render its defense difficult but, by the end of June, almost continuous daylight in the Arctic zone made the task of the German hunters much easier. The convoy had been provided with the strongest protection possible. The close escort comprised two submarines and 19 other vessels, including destroyers, antiaircraft ships, trawlers, corvettes, and minesweepers, all under the command of one of Pound's former midshipmen, Captain Jack Broome. Three destroyers and four cruisers, two of which were American, made up the close covering force. Tovey, who was in command of the distant covering force, had assigned his heavy force to positions northeast of Jan Mayen Island, away from German air attack but in a position to move quickly into the scene of action should major German vessels take to the high seas.

Early in 1942, Hitler feared a British landing in Norway and believed the victory depended on the halting of Allied shipping. At the time, Bismarck's sister ship, Tirpitz, was ready for action, and consequently, Hitler ordered the battleship to sail for Trondheim. She was located there a week later by the British cryptanalysts at Bletchley Park. Earlier in the war, they had deciphered the top-secret system for coded signals transmitted between German naval units and bases.

Hitler reasoned that with Tirpitz stationed there she would be available to counter any British thrust and, if an opportunity occurred, could attack any unprotected Russian-bound merchant convoy. It was evident to him that at the very least, her presence in Norwegian waters would pose an immense problem to the British Admiralty. In this assumption he was correct. Two days after locating the Tirpitz, Churchill, who had followed the affair with his customary interest in naval matters, declared that the destruction or even crippling of this ship seemed of greatest naval importance, there being no other comparable target.

Pound telephoned Tovey on his flagship, Duke of York, at Scapa Flow in the middle of June. Tovey recalled that to his dismay, Pound mentioned that, under certain circumstances, the only course of action might be to order the convoy to scatter so as to prevent its annihilation by Tirpitz. The effect of such an order was for the convoy's ships to abandon their close and disciplined formation and proceed on separate, predetermined, and diverging courses to their individual destinations. It had only been carried out on one occasion, in 1940, when neither enemy aircraft nor submarines had been involved, and the ships had had a vast area in which to disperse and hide.

In the Arctic waters where strong enemy aircraft and submarine forces would be brought into play, the close escort would be more or less powerless to protect their charges once they had scattered, while the area in which they could disperse and hide was much more restricted because of the ice edge and the Norwegian coast. It had been repeatedly proved that even the most weakly escorted convoy stood a better chance if it maintained its cohesion and formation in the face of submarine and air attack. Tovey, therefore, was horrified when Pound seemed to envisage abandoning the convoy and described the proposal as "sheer bloody murder." Tovey's tactics were to use the convoy, with its rich prize of merchantmen, as a fat bait to lure Tirpitz onto the high seas and confront her with the guns of his battle fleet.

The curtain was again hoisted for another naval drama, this time in the Arctic theater, in which PQ 17 was the target for a trial of naval power and an intellectual contest between the opposing naval leaders, Grossadmiral Erich Raeder and Pound. The stage was set for a naval chess match to be played out in the ice-cold Barents Sea by two grand masters. What Raeder did not know was that Pound's mental capacity, in terms of his alertness, cold calculation, and analysis, was waning. What Pound did not know was that Raeder's hands were tied by Hitler who had not forgotten the British massacre of Tirpitz's sister ship in 1941. In fact, Hitler had not been informed by Raeder of Bismarck's sortie onto the high seas and he would not let Tirpitz sail under any circumstances until the whereabouts of the aircraft carrier Victorious in Tovey's force could be ascertained.

A Naval Chess Match

The first six days of PQ 17's voyage were uneventful. The distant drone of German reconnaissance aircraft circling over the convoy beyond the reach of the antiaircraft ships was like the overture to a play. The curtain rose temporarily on the evening of July 2 when the convoy was attacked by Heinkel torpedo bombers. However, no hits were scored, and one of the bombers was shot down.

The first casualty occurred on July 4 when a Heinkel sunk an American freighter; this did not deter other American ships from flying all the Stars and Stripes they could muster in celebration of the 166th anniversary of American independence. At around 8:00 pm there was another attack by Heinkels, with two convoy casualties and two torpedo bombers shot down. The rescue ships stayed behind to pick up the crews and then hurried ahead to positions in the trail of the convoy, where spirits ran high with a feeling of pride and achievement. PQ 17 was by then well past the halfway mark without a single submarine attack, while the efforts of the Luftwaffe had not been all that impressive.

There were only 800 miles to go and the danger of further attacks receded with every passing hour. To the close escort commander, it seemed unlikely that Tirpitz, the "big bad wolf," would stick her neck out Bismarck-fashion. With confidence he wrote in his diary that at this stage he reckoned the convoy could get anywhere as long as the ammunition lasted.

In the meantime, Raeder, realizing that Hitler's fears would threaten any operation by his surface units against PQ 17, ordered Tirpitz to sail from Trondheim to Altenfiord, an anchorage near the northernmost tip of Norway. There she anchored and was joined on July 4 by the heavy cruiser Hipper, the pocket battleship Scheer, and several destroyers.

Over the next 24 hours, while Raeder was pinioned by a hesitant Führer and the surface raiders remained at anchor, the naval chess match was changed by Pound in favor of his opponents. The important information that Tirpitz had entered the Altenfiord on July 4 was delivered to Pound on the evening of the same day via the Operational Intelligence Centre (OIC). The information came from Bletchley Park where the cryptographers had broken the German naval cipher settings for the 24-hour period ending at noon that day. It caused Pound to visit the OIC where he was reassured by Paymaster Commander Norman Denning, chief intelligence officer for German main surface units, that Tirpitz and Hipper had indeed joined Scheer in Altenfiord that morning. They had not, therefore, proceeded directly from Trondheim toward the convoy, and Pound was assured that there was no positive information that Tirpitz had left Altenfiord.

A Disastrous Decision

Pound was not a frequent visitor to OIC and did not seem to have understood the weakness as well as the strengths of special intelligence. Unfortunately, Pound did not ask Denning for detailed reasons why he could state that the German ships remained at anchor. In fact, Denning as well as his superior, Rear Admiral Jock Clayton, director of OIC, and Professor F.H. Hinsley, cryptanalyst in the naval section at Bletchley Park, were all convinced that Tirpitz had not sailed again, due to lack of positive radio reports from the Norwegian underground, the absence of enemy navy signals that always occurred when big ships went to sea, and also by the lack of reports from their own submarines in the area.

After visiting Denning, Pound paid a short visit to the U-boat tracking room and then returned to his own office and called a staff meeting. The circumstances of the meeting were etched in the memory of one officer: ". . . a very tired-looking Dudley Pound sitting gazing in a mesmerized fashion at a small scale chart of the Barents Sea area, calculating with a pair of dividers where the Tirpitz could be at the time." Pound then asked each officer in turn what he would do under the circumstances, and all but one said that the convoy should not be dispersed. Pound then leaned back in his chair and closed his eyes, causing one officer to whisper irreverently, "Look, Father's fallen asleep." After half a minute, Pound opened his eyes and announced, "The convoy is to be dispersed."

Clayton, who had attended the meeting, was depressed when he returned to OIC, as was Denning when he learned the news. He had just received a decrypted enemy signal informing the German U-boats in the vicinity of the convoy that German surface units were not operating in the area. In light of this additional intelligence, Denning persuaded Clayton to go back to Pound and try to change his mind. With great moral courage, Clayton did so but was unsuccessful. Pound told him that the signals had been sent and had probably been acted upon and, in any case, the matter had been decided. By countermanding the order at the time of Clayton's visit, Pound could have prevented the dispersal of convoy PQ 17. Within the next few hours, the impact of his signals on the events in the Barents Sea became irreversible.

It remains an unanswered question whether Pound notified Churchill of his decision on that evening. If he did, it may explain why he also ignored Clayton's suggestion, Tovey's protests, Denning's intelligence information, and the negative attitude towards convoy dispersal expressed by his own staff. A disastrous mistake in handling intelligence reports had again been committed at the British Admiralty. But it was not a fault in passing on important information, as had been the case 26 years earlier. This time it was a complete failure by Pound to comprehend the weight and magnitude of the available intelligence, a failure that inevitably was to result in the most disastrous consequences for hundreds of men, but not for Pound himself.

Disastrous Consequences of Failure of Comprehension

Pound's signal, sent from an armchair some 2,000 miles away, exploded in the hands of the commander of the close escort force, Captain Broome, who either had to obey or ignore it. Broome afterward reproached himself and has repeatedly stated that to his dying regret he obeyed the signal to scatter the convoy. But what else could he do? It was a clear-cut order, it could not be discussed, and it originated from the top. As the flag captain to the commander of the distant covering force said when discussing the tragedy shortly afterward, "Not even Lord Nelson could have ignored a series of signals like those."

Pound's order to scatter convoy PQ 17, which was obeyed by the astonished and reluctant captains of the merchant ships and escort vessels, triggered a sequence of events that resulted in a terrible massacre. By ordering the dispersal, Pound had placed the individual merchant ships at the mercy of the German submarines and Luftwaffe who showed no mercy. They picked the ships off almost at will, one by one, turning the waters of the Barents Sea into a shooting gallery. Altogether 23 ships in the convoy were sunk in the cold Arctic water, 10 by U-boats and 13 by the Luftwaffe.

Churchill called the tragedy one of the most melancholy naval episodes of the whole war, while Stalin asked Churchill if the British navy had any sense of glory. Only 11 merchant ships finally reached Archangel. Of 4,246 vehicles, 594 tanks, and 297 aircraft carried by the convoy, 3,350, 430, and 210, respectively, were lost, as well as 99,316 tons of general cargo, including crated vehicles, radar sets, food, steelplate, and ammunition. Worst of all, 146 men died, many of them a painful death.

There are many gruesome accounts, such as those given by survivors from the British merchant ship Hartlebury, which had almost reached Novaya Zemlya when she was torpedoed by Commander Günther La Baume's U-355 on July 7: Soon after the third torpedo struck, the ship broke into three sections, and began her final plunge. In a lifeboat that was so overcrowded that there was no hope of making it seaworthy, the men saw another one from the crew on their dying ship. It was the second officer, Harold Spence, who had been left on the middle section of the sinking wreck. They saw him stripping off his lifejacket, his coat, and finally his cap. He had resigned himself to his fate. As the merchant ship finally plunged groaning beneath the waves, the last sight of him was a figure waving to them from the bridge. Then the waves poured over him. Spence had been married just 10 days before Hartlebury had sailed from Sunderland on her last voyage.

Another eyewitness gave the following account:

> "Geoffrey Dixon had not been in the lifeboat more than an hour before he started going off his head; he began to rave that they had no hope, and they were all going to die. He had been sitting up to his armpits in water. After a time, he began ducking his head underwater, trying to drown himself; the others had restrained him, but after a while he had seemed to drift off to sleep. Gradually his eyes had opened and from his awkward position the third officer guessed that he was dead. He and another seaman lifted the unfortunate Able Seaman over the side of the boat into the sea, and pushed him gently under.
>
> "We had only been about an hour in the overcrowded lifeboat when Geoffrey Dixon died. After Dixon's death, the men began to die one by one. Most of those who died early were men from the engine-room who had rushed on deck when the ship was torpedoed dressed only in short-sleeved undershirts. The next to die was our radio officer Sibitt. He lost his nerves, giving up all hope and just falling asleep not to wake up anymore. Within the first four hours, 15 men in our

boat just went away the same way. We were only five of us left when John Storey, the last man from the engine-room to be alive, without saying a word jumped overboard. With powerful strokes he swam into the bank of mist. With weak voices we tried to call him back but he wouldn't listen to us. And we were so apathetic that we didn't even look after him as he disappeared forever."

For those who survived the enemy's attack there were dreadful days or weeks in open lifeboats and rafts on the ice-cold Arctic Sea, a frightful experience only to be followed, in many instances, by years in German prison camps. Many seamen were severely frostbitten, and even those not captured by the Germans were faced with a terrible existence.

The head of the British naval mission in Moscow visited the Russian field "hospitals" in the Kola peninsula and was horrified. He saw the most ghastly clinical problems, including two young British seamen who had lost all their limbs from frostbite. In the airless, squalid wards, boards nailed over the windows as a blackout were a permanent fixture, allowing little ventilation for the varied smells. From 7 o'clock in the morning until 11 at night, loudspeakers blared unceasingly in Russian. Drugs were short and pain regarded with oriental indifference by surgeons and physicians. Dull, monotonous food did nothing to comfort men lying in fear and pain, unable to make their simplest needs or symptoms known. British surgeons did what they could, but, owing to professional jealousy, were only permitted to visit the patients and attend operations as laymen. They were neither consulted nor allowed to advise.

No information regarding convoy PQ 17 reached either the British or the American public before 1945. A captured American seaman, put under lock and key in the Marlag-Milag Nord Prison Camp on Lüneburg Heath in Germany, wrote a brief account of the disaster to his wife in the United States. His letter, forwarded by the Red Cross out of Germany, was censored, and his description of how "the naval escort left the convoy and we were told to split up and make port best we could alone," and of how "the entire convoy was defenseless and sunk by bombers" as a result, was excised by American censors.

On the Responsibility for the PQ 17 Disaster

On July 28 an inquiry into the PQ 17 disaster, ordered by Churchill, took place in a room in the House of Commons. Apart from Pound, Eden (the foreign secretary), Maisky (the Russian ambassador), A.V. Alexander (the first lord of the Admiralty), a Russian admiral, Kharlamov, and his assistant were present. Pound was invited by Eden to give an explanation, but before he could do so, he was interrupted by Maisky who asked when the next PQ convoy would sail. Admiral Kharlamov then started to criticize Pound's order to scatter convoy PQ 17 to which Pound reacted strongly. As his face grew redder and redder, he retorted, "That order was given by me! Me! What else should have been done?" Alexander then apologized for Pound's disastrous decision, whereupon Maisky ingratiatingly commented that, "even British admirals make mistakes." With this Pound grew even more furious and exclaimed, "Tomorrow I shall ask the Prime Minister to appoint you First Sea Lord instead of myself."

Four days later, Pound told the war cabinet that he had ordered convoy PQ 17 to scatter because he had learned that Tirpitz had eluded the patrolling British submarines off North Cape and could be in a position to attack it on the morning of July 5. The existence of such precise intelligence has, however, not been confirmed by postwar research.

When Broome, commanding the destroyer Keppel in the close convoy escort that ceased to exist on the evening of July 4, finally returned, he received a message announcing a personal visit by the first lord on docking. Broome reckoned that the unsolved nightmare—Why had convoy PQ 17 been ordered to scatter?—might be explained. When the lord inspected the ship's company he was asked down to Broome's cabin. As Broome later described, "The moment of truth seemed near. When we were alone I asked him point blank: 'Why was PQ 17 scattered?' All I remember about the answer I got was that it was no answer, or moment of truth. My question was precisely what he had come, armed with evasive politics, to decry." Broome's conclusion was that, had the Admiralty's conscience about PQ 17 been clear, he would never have had the doubtful pleasure of the first lord's visit to his ship.

The passage in Churchill's postwar memoirs about the PQ 17 tragedy was ghosted by George Allen, a captain in the naval staff at the Admiralty during the war. Allen had declared that Churchill himself inserted a most unlikely explanation for Pound's disastrous signals, namely that Pound signaled the cruiser escort—half of which was American—to withdraw, and the convoy to scatter, so as not to endanger the American ships. Nothing in the naval records suggests that this was the case. On occasion, Churchill was wont to invent extenuating circumstances to mitigate the errors of his protégés, and he was trying to make excuses for Pound.

At the time, Churchill probably did not know that it was Pound who alone and against all advice made the fatal decision in July 1942. When Allen informed Churchill in 1949 that his research among the official papers and his interviews with naval staff officers revealed that Pound was responsible for the decision, he could see "real pain and grief written across Churchill's face; he had not known about it." Accordingly, in Churchill's *The Hinge of Fate* he stated, "So strictly was the secret of these orders being sent on the first sea lord's authority guarded by the Admiralty, that it was not until after the war that I learned the facts."

Dudley Pound's Brain Failure

Pound certainly suffered from two types of brain failure: the first mental exhaustion and the second brain destruction due to the infiltration of a glioma in the left cerebral hemisphere. He was 62 years old when summoned home from the Mediterranean in 1939 to the Admiralty to become first sea lord. His partnership with Churchill turned out to be unlucky for him: the late hours kept by Churchill and his lack of consideration toward Pound and his hardworking staff must have contributed greatly to the strain on Pound.

The secret of Churchill's stamina lay in his habit of undressing and taking an afternoon nap in bed, exploiting "to the full my happy gift of falling almost immediately into deep sleep. By this means I was able to press a day and a half's work into one," he explained.

Churchill regularly worked into the night until two or three in the morning and was ready for more between eight and nine. When he became prime minister, he continued to keep in direct contact with Pound. His appointee as first lord of the Admiralty, A.V. Alexander, was a weak individual appointed to the Admiralty so as not to interfere too much with the naval side of the war. Consequently, Churchill normally spoke to Pound on the telephone in the early hours of the morning (neither went to bed until around 3:00 am).

And Pound would go along punctiliously to see Alexander to tell him what had happened during the day and what Churchill had said. Certainly Churchill and Pound thought that they could conduct the war at sea far better than anyone else.

For Pound, a mediocre character without Churchill's exceptional capacities, the aforementioned conditions were sooner or later to lead to mental exhaustion. That such was the case is also supported by numerous descriptions that Pound looked more and more tired, old, and at the end of his tether as the war progressed.

An attempt at evaluating more exactly when brain destruction was superimposed on mental exhaustion becomes difficult or impossible since neither a tumor biopsy nor an autopsy was performed. Nevertheless, there is no reason to question the diagnosis of a malignant glioma in the left cerebral hemisphere that was arrived at independently by two experienced and distinguished neurospecialists.

Pound's main trouble in the end was his increasing dysphasia. He did not show overt clinical signs of increased intracranial pressure, apart from papilledema at a late stage of his illness. The fact that symptoms of brain destruction dominated those of increased intracranial pressure indicates that the growth may have originated in, and been mainly confined to, deeper structures such as the basal ganglia.

One may speculate whether Pound suffered for several years from a low-grade astrocytoma that finally developed into a fulminant glioblastoma multiform. If so, the insidious symptoms of brain failure with a decrease in mental alertness and capacity for comprehension and logical thought, observed by several distinguished naval officers, could be ascribed to an initially slow-growing and destructive tumor.

Although a final assessment of the influence of the different factors behind Pound's brain failure during his last years cannot be settled more exactly, it seems justifiable to conclude that it was not an admiral with a fully fit mind who led the British navy in the years 1940 to 1943.

Churchill often remarked that Pound was one of the three men whose companionship meant most to him, the others being the South African prime minister, General Jan Smuts, and Lord Beaverbrook. Pound's death on the anniversary of Trafalgar greatly distressed Churchill, who was visibly sad after his close friend's death. Had Pound not been held in such high esteem by Churchill, possibly other admirals would have forced him to consult a physician at an early stage. Had he then been forced to retire, fatal decisions would not have been made, and Spence, Dixon, Sibitt, and Storey, and many more would have escaped an agonizing death or otherwise horrible and grueling experience.

Perhaps Churchill simply kept Pound so long in office in order to be able to intervene in the events related to his cherished and glorious Royal Navy without opposition (from an acquiescent and sick first sea lord)? There was a similar situation with Roosevelt and his first secretary of the navy, Claude Swanson. Swanson was an invalid (like Roosevelt), but also a weak and ineffective man. Roosevelt kept him on until Swanson finally died in office, so that in the interim Roosevelt could run his beloved navy as he chose.

On the other hand, Pound's American opposite, Fleet Admiral Ernest King (Fig 31), was a strong man, who became the first American naval officer to wear five stars and carry the rank and title of Fleet Admiral. Only two years before King was appointed to commander-in-chief of all naval operations by Roosevelt, it was said that he drank too much, chased other men's wives, and made too many enemies. Why, then, did Roosevelt elevate him to become the most powerful naval officer in history? King had a simple answer, "When the Big Guys get into trouble, they send for the sons-of-bitches."

Selected References

1. Accoce R, Rentchnick P. *Ces malades qui nous gouvernement.* City, France: Editions Stock; 1976.

2. Beesly P. *Very Special Admiral: The Life of Admiral JH Godfrey.* London, England: Hamish Hamilton; 1980.

3. Beesly P. *Very Special Intelligence: The Story of the Admiralty's Operational Intelligence Centre 1939-1945.* London, England: Hamish Hamilton; 1977.

4. Broome J. *Convoy Is to Scatter.* London, England: William Kimber; 1972.

5. Broome J. I am ready and willing to go back. In: Winton J, ed. *Freedom's Battle: The War at Sea 1939-1945.* 1st vol. London, England: Hutchinson of London; 1967.

6. Bryant A. *The Turn of the Tide—1939-1943: A Study Based on the Diaries and Autobiographical Notes of Field Marshal The Viscount Alanbrooke.* London, England: Collins; 1957.

7. Buell TB. *Master of Sea Power: A Biography of Fleet Admiral Ernest J. King.* Boston, Mass: Little, Brown & Co; 1980.

8. Butler JRM. *Lord Lothian (Philip Kerr) 1882-1940.* London, England: Macmillan; 1960.

9. Churchill WS. *Memories of the Second World War: Closing the Ring.* 5th vol. London, England: Cassell & Co; 1948.

10. Churchill WS. *Memories of the Second World War: The Hinge of Fate.* 4th vol. London, England: Cassell & Co; 1948.

11. Edwards K. *Men of Action.* London, England: Collins; 1943.

12. Irving D. *The Destruction of Convoy PQ 17.* London, England: Cassell & Co; 1968.

13. Joel D. *Admiral of the Fleet Sir Dudley Pound.* Available in: Imperial War Museum, London, England: 1970. Leaflet.

14. Karweina G. *Geleitzug PQ 17: Ein Tatsachenbericht.* Hamburg, Germany: Mosaik Verlag; 1964.

15. Kennedy L. *Menace: The Life and Death of the Tirpitz.* Devon, England: Wheaton & Co; 1979.

16. Kennedy L. *Pursuit: The Chase and Sinking of the Bismarck.* London, England: Collins; 1974.

17. Liddel Hart BH. *The Memoirs of Captain Liddell Hart.* 2nd vol. London, England: Cassel & Co; 1965:263.

18. Ljunggren B. The sleepy sea lord who was Churchill's friend. *Surg Neurol.* 1982;18:307-319.

19. Maisky I. Memoirs. In: *Novye Mir.* 7th vol. Moscow, USSR; 1965.

20. Marder A. Winston is back: Churchill at the Admiralty, 1939-1940. In: Wallace-Hadrill JM, Roberts JM, eds. *The English Historical Review.* 1972;(suppl 5).

21. McLachlan D. *Room 39: Naval Intelligence in Action 1939-45.* London, England: Weidenfelt & Nicholson; 1968.

22. Moran CMW. *Winston Churchill: The Struggle for Survival 1940-1965.* London, England: Constable & Co; 1966.

23. Petrow R. *The Bitter Years: The Invasion and Occupation of Denmark and Norway April 1940-May 1945.* London, England: Hodder & Stoughton; 1975.

24. Roskill SW. *Churchill and the Admirals.* London, England: Collins; 1977.

25. Roskill SW. Information in file concerning Sir Dudley Pound. Available in: Archives Centre, Churchill College, Cambridge, England.

26. Roskill SW. *The War at Sea.* 1st-3rd vols. London, England: Her Majesty's Stationery Office; 1956-1961.

27. von Müllenheim-Rechberg B. *Battleship Bismarck: A Survivor's Story.* London, England: Bodley Head Ltd; 1980.

28. Weaver HJ. *Nightmare at Scapa Flow: The Truth About the Sinking of HMS Royal Oak.* Oxfordshire, England: Cresstelles Co; 1980.

29. Winterbotham FW. *The Ultra Secret.* London, England: Weidenfelt & Nicolson; 1974.

Chapter 9

The Good Old Method of the Nail

Reprinted by permission of the publisher from *Surgical Neurology*.

In 1976, two unusual cases of nails driven into the brain under inhumane circumstances were described in *Surgical Neurology*. Those cases were referred to as being unique.

A similar case treated in the author's clinic prompted a review of the literature on this subject. This method of killing a person is found in the Bible, where it is described in the Book of Judges. The method recurs in the wave of witch persecutions in England during the Middle Ages, when professional "prickers" stuck pins into suspected spots on the body, including the scalp, to find out the possessor's eventual branding by Satan.

Furthermore, this method of killing a person was depicted by Sweden's best-known author, August Strindberg (1849-1912), in his novel *By the Open Sea*, in which the author refers to this violent act as "the good old method of the nail"—suggesting that the method has been known for a long time in our society. In addition, this method also has been described by other Scandinavian authors of repute during the last century.

Case Report

On October 20, 1973, the ambulance in one of the big cities in Sweden was called for an emergency case. Arriving at a tenement in an older estate, the ambulance men found signs of a fight (Fig 33) and an unconscious, beaten woman, who was immediately transported to the emergency department of a nearby hospital. On admission there, she was comatose and had a right hemiparesis as well as deviation conjugée to the left. When the temporary head bandage was removed, her calvarium presented as "a soup of more or less" loose cutaneous strips and blood clots with still bleeding tattered and torn vessels. Blood transfusions were instantly given and X-rays of the skull were made.

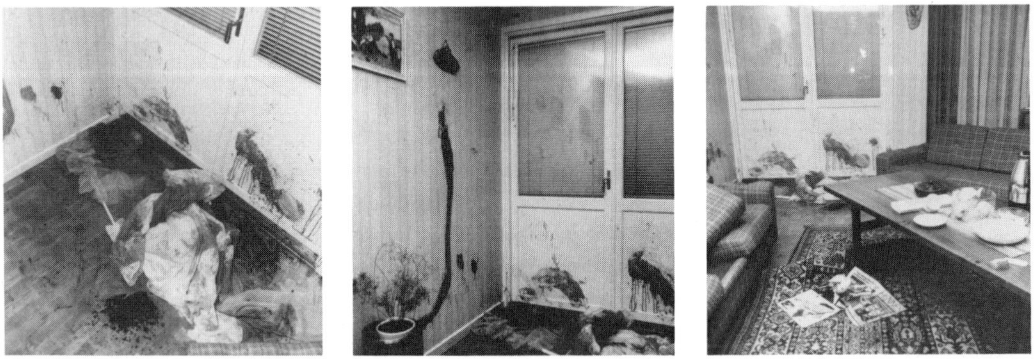

Figure 33: *Interior of the tenement where the act of violence took place. (Photographs taken by the police.)*

At that time, the police telephoned the hospital to say that they had seized the patient's husband, who already admitted that he had assaulted his wife with a hammer and an awl in order to "exorcise the evil soul that had taken its place in her head." The husband had especially bought a set of tools, including the awl, at a cost of three and a half Swedish crowns (about 75 U.S. cents) (Fig 34). The police stated that they had found the hammer but not the awl at the scene of the crime.

Soon thereafter, the X-ray examination of the skull was completed with a most surprising result. There were multiple slightly depressed skull fractures in the midline of the forehead and an 11 cm long metallic awl completely inside the skull and through both cerebral hemispheres (Fig 35). The patient was immediately transferred to the author's clinic.

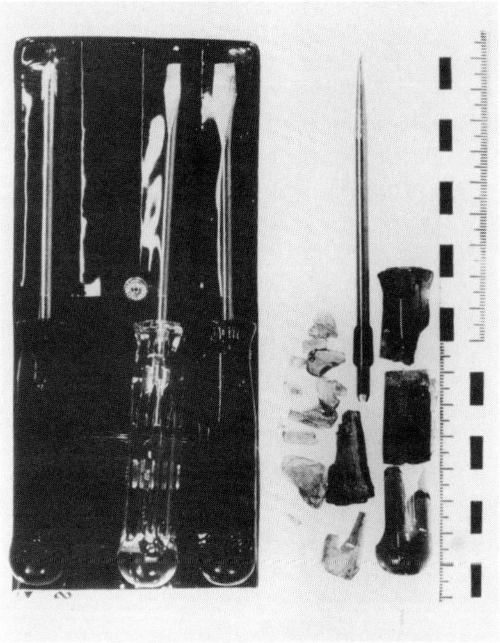

Figure 34: *To the left, a set of chisels with the set from which the man had chosen the awl. To the right, the awl that was used in the actual case. The shaft is broken; the different parts of the shaft were found by the police on the floor at the place of the deed. The peak of the awl had become slightly bent when the man had driven it into the base of the skull.*

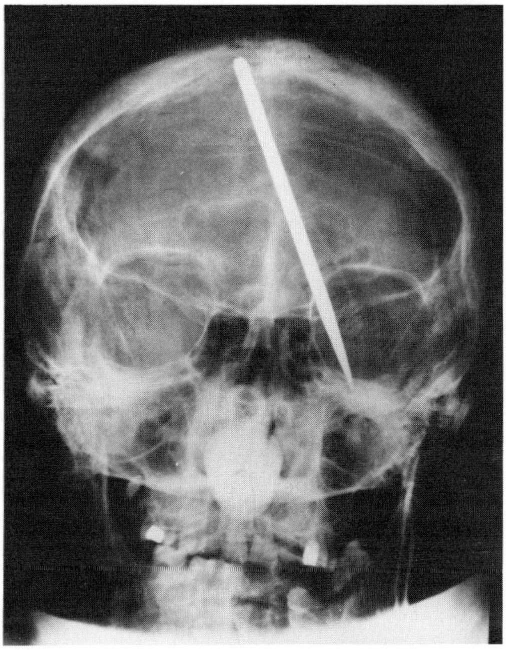

Figure 35: *Frontal X-ray film of the skull with the awl driven in from the right side close to the superior sagittal sinus and through falx cerebri. The peak of the awl rests on the petrous pyramid on the left side. The exact length of the awl was 11.2 cm and the diameter at the base, 4.5 mm.*

On the evening of admission, under endotracheal anesthesia, the entrance/opening for the awl was exposed. The end of the chisel was exactly at the level of the skull bone so that it had to be extracted via a separate burr hole quite close to the point of entrance of the awl. The extraction was carried out without difficulty. The superior sagittal sinus fortunately was intact; the awl had been driven into the brain close to its lateral wall. Finally, the widespread scalp lesions were treated. Three weeks later the patient left the clinic in fairly good condition.

When seen several years later, the patient appeared to be in good general condition, behaving normally, walking with a stick and having only a slight right hemiparesis. She has had no epileptic seizures. Her husband has received treatment at a mental hospital for a schizophrenia with paranoid delusions.

Review of the Literature

The technique of driving a nail into the brain in order to kill a person is already described in the Old Testament in the Book of Judges 4:21-22, and the text goes as follows:

> "Then Jael, Heber's wife, took a nail of the tent, and took a hammer in her hand, and went softly unto Sisera, and smote the nail into his temples, and fastened it into the ground: for he was asleep and weary. So he died.
>
> "And, behold, as Barak pursued Sisera, Jael came out to meet him, and said unto him, come, and I will shew thee the man whom thou seekest. And when he came into her tent, behold, Sisera lay dead, and the nail was in his temples."

In *The Canterbury Tales*—the grand work that made his name immortal—Geoffrey Chaucer (the greatest poet in England before Shakespeare) described different ways wives have put their husbands to death. The prologue to "The Tale of the Wyf of Bathe" ("Wife of Bath's Preamble") deals with a wife, who on a journey tells her fellow travelers about her marriages (she has survived five men). She tells: When in disputatious mood, one of her husbands grew familiar with the habit of reading aloud from books concerning wives who had been abusive and tiresome in general or who had maltreated or even poisoned and killed their husbands. He read aloud about a wife who was not afraid of killing her husband in his own bed so that she could then devote herself to amorous excesses with her lover in the same room.

It then reads, "And some han [have] drive nayles in hir [their] brayn Whyl that they slepte, and thus they han them slayn" or in another version "And some han dreuyn [driven] nayles in here brayne Whyle that they slep and thus han hem slayne." The wife of Bath reins her husband in and lectures him soundly for his bad habits of such readings, whereupon peace settles upon their home.

During the Middle Ages, there was another reason for driving nails into people's skulls. At that time some people were of the opinion that the witches were marked by some mole, birthmark, or scar, supposedly indicating the possessor's branding by Satan. Generally, as a preliminary to being searched for the devil's mark, the suspect was completely shaved, to reveal anything hidden by hair. If a suspected witch had no such obvious marks, she might still have invisible marks, discovered only by pricking.

The operations were performed by special "prickers," who used certain instruments especially designed for this purpose. The "prickers" drove a long pin into the spot suspected to represent a devil's mark or *Stigmata diaboli* or *Sigillum diaboli* and often located on the scalp.

It was regarded as conclusive that it was a devil's mark and that the possessor was a witch if no pain was felt and no blood ran out when the long pin was driven into the person under suspicion. It seems possible that the "prickers" sometimes perforated the skull so that the pins were driven into the brain.

In the book *At the Open Sea*, published 1890 (English translation 1913), August Strindberg, the famous Swedish author, describes a case that is briefly reported here:

A fisheries inspector by the name of Borg stayed for some time on an island in the archipelago of Stockholm in order to improve the fishery. He boarded and lodged with a custom house attendant named Vestman. Here lived also Vestman's brother, who was a preventive officer. The wife of the custom house attendant lived in bigamy, i.e. the brother-in-law was her lover.

One evening, Vestman's maid came running to Borg and begged him to visit her mistress, who was dying. Borg hurried to the custom house and was received by the two brothers with a suspicious politeness. But he said nothing, asked no questions. He saw at once that she was dead. He could tell from the contracted muscles of her face that she had died by violence. When he saw that her hair was carefully combed across the part, he had no doubt that the good old method of the nail had been chosen. But he was determined to make Vestman speak first.

Vestman believed that he did not need to be on his guard and said, "You might certify, mister, that she is dead, then we could bury her straight away; no need to tell you that poor people like we can't afford to send for a doctor." Borg had heard enough. He looked at Vestman, who was now perfectly calm, and whispered, "Where's the hammer?"

Vestman took a step or two back, as if he meant to throw himself upon his opponent and strangle him. Borg disarmed him by a look. The man stood before him, shaking. "He has no idea where the hammer is, but I know where the nail can be found," continued Borg, imperturbably. "Oh! you self-sufficient donkeys who cannot invent anything new but, like children, always hide in the same spot when they play hide and seek. Surely this nailing of the brain was invented in the Middle Ages by a priest or a nobleman and has only now reached the lower classes, instead of being, as is always stated, a proof of their cunning."

The next author to describe the method is the Finnish author Johannes Linnankoski (1869-1913). In *Taistelu Heikkilläu talosta* (*The Struggle for the Farm of Heikkilä*) he spins the following story:

Christmas was over and the next-door neighbor to the farm of Heikkilä, the blacksmith, held a big feast for all his neighbors. Then—in the midst of a raving polka—all of a sudden the door was pulled up and on the doorstep stood the master of Heikkilä: "The inmates of Heikkilä must come home at once!" He did not succeed in getting anything more out from his mouth. In the next moment he was away. Everyone understood that something particular had happened or was happening so everyone began to move towards the farm of Heikkilä.

The master led them straight to the parlor of the landlady where the mistress was lying pale and undressed in her bed, her face outward, with both hands to her chest, as if she had had heart pains. Now the master told how he had woke up in his room from an outcry and moaning. He had hurried to the mistress but got so afraid when seeing her that he had left and hurried to the feast to call for help.

Everyone understood that she must have died shortly before in some kind of a heart attack. The neighbors left in low spirits and the women of the farm began to clean up the dead body. The master was present everywhere, helped to raise and turn the body and hold the head of his dead wife when the hair was combed. The servants were struck with wonder at the humanity and goodness that their master showed, for he was known to be an evil man. The funeral was as splendid and grand as befitted such a farm and such a person, who was honored and esteemed by everyone—as distinguished from her husband, the master, who had always seemed to be beset by the devil.

Twenty years had passed since the death of the mistress when a man came visiting the parsonage and said he had an important message. His appearance bore witness of mental excitement. The parson, though not already dressed, issued orders for the man to be shown into his office. And there the man began talking hastily, with quaking voice and his face distorted by nervous twitchings. He had known the mistress of Heikkilä farm very well. All color vanished from the man's face and he shivered. "It was, yes, I am sure that it was a . . . nail of iron. A nail of iron . . . ? Yes!"

The parson remained silent for a moment. "Well, to tell the truth, I must confess that I myself was somewhat suspicious at that time. That was just the reason why I went to see the body—but the dead mistress rested so calmly and peacefully in her coffin and I could discover no trace of violence. Now I can understand the hint of God the Almighty. Go, my sorely tried friend, to the farm-hands' quarters and order them to put the horse between the shafts—we are both of us driving to the head of the country constabulary."

The grave was opened the same day. "In the backhead of the dead body, just below the knot of hair a thick, six inch ironnail was found. It had been driven right into the brain and so deep that the nailhead could scarcely be discovered." Soon thereafter the farmer of Heikkilä farm was thrown into irons and sentenced for his old crime.

Among the most successful books ever to have appeared in Sweden are Vilhelm Moberg's (1898-1973) great trilogy of novels about the Swedish emigrants to America in the 19th century. In the opening volume, *The Emigrants*, Moberg tells how a handful of persecuted and poverty-stricken men and women left Sweden a century ago and faced the Atlantic, believing that beyond it they would find a free, happy country of opportunity. On their way to the ship, the farmer, Jonas Petter, sat on the coachbox. While driving by a fine gray manor house on top of a knoll and with the name of Galtakullen, Vilhelm Moberg lets Jonas Petter tell the following story:

It was said that the farmer of Galtakullen could never satisfy his wife, Lotta Andersdotter, in bed; she was that kind of woman whom no man could please however much he worked and tried. Now she wanted to exchange her husband for the enlisted man of the village, a strong, bed-worthy man. And the soldier was tempted by the promise that he was to be the farmer of Galtakullen.

One night when her husband was sleeping soundly, Lotta Andersdotter got out of bed and went to the toolbox for a hammer and a five-inch spike. With the hammer she drove the spike full length into the skull of her sleeping husband. He never awakened—unless it were in heaven or hell. Some blood splurted out of the hole in his head, but the murderess dried it off and left the nailhead well covered by her husband's hair.

She then announced that her husband had died from a stroke; as people knew, he had been somewhat ailing lately. A grand funeral was held. The widow wanted to show that she mourned her husband deeply, and she cried profusely and bitterly at the graveside. No one suspected her of a crime.

As soon as her widow year was up, she married the soldier. He, in his turn, died after 10 years of wedded life from somewhat more natural causes than the first husband: people said from overwork in bed.

The housewife of Galtakullen remained the same craving woman; she was about to take a third husband, but he became frightened of her and changed his mind before it was too late. He is supposed to have said that the widow at Galtakullen was almost as much man as woman, that she had the organs of both sexes—though no one could be sure of this. After two marriages she sat, a widow, on her farm for the rest of her life.

Then, 30 years after her first husband's sudden death, the gravedigger was one day opening a new grave in the churchyard. While digging, he got hold of a skull on his spade. He usually paid no attention to a skull, big or small, any more than a potato picker looks at his potatoes; for human skulls grow in a churchyard as profusely as tubers in a field. But this skull was different: a long rusty-red spike hung rattling inside it. The gravedigger carried his find to the dean and pointed out to him where he had found the skull. The dean looked up his records and made sure of who had once been buried in that place. He then tied the skull up in a piece of black cloth, took it under his arm, and went directly to Galtakullen. The widow was at home, he handed her the parcel, and said, "Here comes your first husband to visit you; he wishes to speak about the nail in his head. Later you can come to me and speak about your wretched soul." With this the dean went home.

The following day, the widow Lotta Andersdotter went to the parsonage and confessed her crime. And in the evening that same day, she hanged herself in the milk cellar of the farm. "Right in there, in that gray house up there," concluded Jonas Petter.

Chinese Nail Murders

The nail murder is one of the most famous motifs in Chinese crime literature. The oldest source is quoted in the casebook *T'ang-yin pi-shih*, where the solution is ascribed to Yen Tsun, a clever judge.

The point of these stories is always the same: the judge is baffled by the fact that although there are strong reasons for suspecting the wife, the body of the husband shows no signs of violence. The final discovery of the nail is elaborated in various ways.

The oldest version said that Yen Tsun found it because he noted that a swarm of flies congregated on one place on top of the dead man's skull. The latest version occurs in the 18th century Chinese detective novel, *Wu-tse-t'ien-szu-ta-ch'i-an*, published in English in Tokyo under the title *Dee Goong An*; there the judge finally elicits a confession from the guilty widow by staging in the tribunal a scene from hell that makes the woman think she is appearing before the Judge of the Nether World.

In 1881, Stent recorded another version under the title "The Double Nail Murders" in volume 10 of the *China Review*: When the coroner fails to discover any trace of violence on the victim's corpse, his own wife suggests to him that he look for a nail. When the judge has convicted the murdered man's widow on this evidence, he also has the coroner's wife brought to him, since her knowledge of such a subtle way of committing a murder seems suspicious to him. It transpires that the coroner is her second husband. The corpse of her first husband is exhumed, and a nail discovered inside the skull. Both women are executed.

Comment

In the literature "the good old method of the nail" has been known for long. The interesting point is that literature knows of no surviving cases. Obviously, all earlier authors who have depicted the method have been of the opinion that nailing of the brain must lead to immediate death. That this need not be the case at all is illustrated by the authentic case report initiating this review.

Selected References

1. Book of Judges 4:21-22.

2. Chaucer G. The tale of the wyf of bathe. In: *Canterbury Tales.* (Chaucer's Society's Publication. 1901;95(1):769-770.) London, England: Kegan Paul, Trench, Trübner & Co; 1901:188.

3. Linnankoski J; Nohrström H, trans. *Taistelu Heikilläu talosta* [in Finnish]. Helsinki, Finland: Holger Schildts Förlagsaktiebolag; 1919:30-71.

4. Ljunggren B, Strömblad LG. The good old method of the nail. *Surg Neurol.* 1977;7:288-292.

5. Moberg Vilhelm; Lannestock G, trans. *The Emigrants* [in Swedish]. Stockholm, Sweden: Albert Bonniers Co; 1969:181-182.

6. Olumide AA, Adeloye A. Unusual cranio-cerebral injuries: report of two cases in Nigerians. *Surg Neurol.* 1976;6:306-308.

7. Rossel HR. *The Encyclopedia of Witchcraft and Demonology.* London, England: Spring Books; 1955:135-137,399-401.

8. Strindberg A; Schleussner E, trans. *By the Open Sea.* New York, NY: Huebsch; 1913:310-312.

9. van Gulik R. *The Chinese Nail Murders.* England: Avon Book Publishing Co; 1961:181-182.